Dominant Health
The Nutrition and Lifestyle Guide to Powerful, Optimum Health

Learn the surprising secrets to

Disease-Proof Your Body

Lose Weight that Stays Off

Look Great Naturally

Stay Young Longer

Eat Well – Cheaply and Easily

By Matthew "Raw Matt" Nailor

Professional Fight Champion,
Lecturer, Formulator of Epic Elixirs,
and Ordained Essene

Edited by anand

Library of Congress Cataloging-in-Publication Data
Nailor, Matthew
Dominant Health: the Nutrition and Lifestyle Guide to Powerful, Optimum Health

Summary: Dominant Health is a collection of studies, research, and practical advice written for the purposes of helping people learn how to stay disease-free, manage their weight healthfully, look great, and stay young longer.

ISBN-13: 978-1977851666 CreateSpace
ISBN- 10: 1977851665

1. Self Help/Personal Transformation
2. Self Help/Motivational
3. Health, Fitness & Dieting/Aging Nutrition & Diets
I. Nailor, Matthew II. Title

Published by Futura House
2620 South Maryland Parkway #345
Las Vegas, NV 89109
Printed in the United States of America
www.futurahouse.com

Cover photo and book design by MM Stratton (megorama.com)
using News Gothic and Garamond ITC fonts.

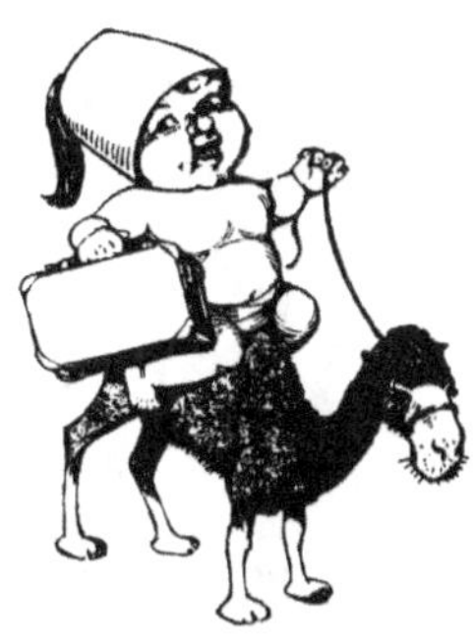

CONTENTS

Health Issues

Technologies

Conclusions

Appendices

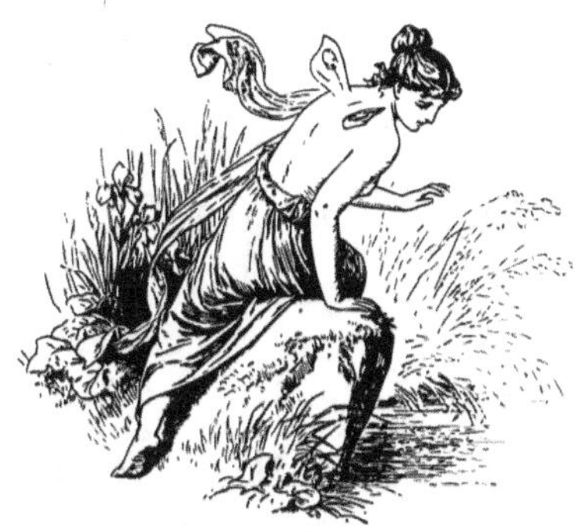

Forward

*"Our Earth has an abundance
of pure and harmless foods
and there is no need for us to partake
of meals for which blood has to be shed
and innocent life sacrificed."*

Pythagoras

I have been privileged to know 'Raw Matt' since the early 2000s. The world is blessed to have such a resourcefully-educated, enthusiastic, and passionate person around. He has influenced countless people to live better lives and inspired many health teachers and coaches to greatness. His wide expanse of knowledge has helped both myself and my husband find healthy ways of being in the world. He specifically was very pivotal in my overcoming an Obsessive-

Compulsive addiction type of disorder, known as Excoriation Disorder, by simply improving my diet. For this I am forever grateful.

Several years after we met, Matthew said he was working on a potential book. He had a bunch of notes outlining his ideas about health from a religious, nutritional and philosophical perspective. I was very keen to read what he had written. At that point they were simply a series of short form essays and random thoughts, along with many copied and pasted articles and quotes from other authors that required they be re-written in Matthew's own voice in order not to un-ethically appropriate them. I eventually offered to help him edit his notes into a proper full-length book.

Matthew wanted to make sure the information got disseminated to as many people as possible without any barriers to sharing the insights he had gathered. The decision was made to offer a downloadable PDF for free on his website.

As the way of the web shall be, the website is no more, and the online version is 'out of print' so to speak.

Flash forward to over a decade later,
I finished writing the books, <u>Kiss Addiction Goodbye</u> and <u>Stop Picking on Me</u>. Each book links addiction and OCD behavior directly to diet and mindfulness. In each of these books, I acknowledged the role that Matthew had played in my own personal recovery.

And I came to think about that 'other' book that was written many years prior, and I was sad to know it was no more to be seen by the world. Since I still had the original source files for the book, I contacted Matthew to see if he would be amenable to putting out a 'non-disappearing' hard copy of the book and he agreed. And so here we are. You have first person access to a truly gifted healer and educator in your hands.

If you are dealing with a condition that is not being successfully treated by the standard mainstream medical community, I invite you to open this book and read the no-nonsense approach that Matthew takes to improving your health. Some of his original words involved more religious tonality to them. These were toned down as to not drive away the atheist or agnostic from reading. I went back and reinstated that language.

I hope that Matthew's words will provide you with great hope for healing, and deep faith for your future.

~anand

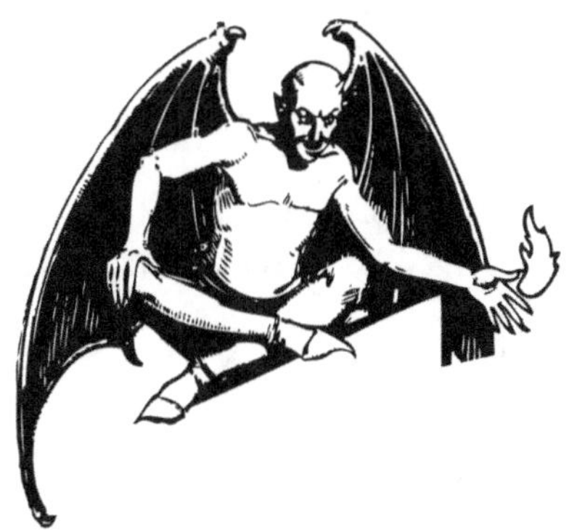

PREFACE

I strive to take my "self" out of the equation in all aspects of my life. I desire to have no desires for I do not wish to be driven by fear on unfulfilled desire. I aspire to live in a present state of mind. This, deep down is what we all must strive for. But we get lost as Satan shrouds our mind with the ego and "self" importance.

Satan is not a physical being with horns and a tail, but rather a manifestation of the mind. His specter works to rob and steal your life. In the Bible, he is called the "Power of Darkness" in Colossians 1:13. Thus, we are to always look towards "Light." When we look away from the light, we see the darkness of our shadow, and there we find illness and sorrow.

When we age, our egos get in the way of true self. They shadow us. We say to ourselves that, "Well, I need to do this, or I am this." We set labels on ourselves that inevitably cause stress and burden in our lives.

Symbiotic Relationships

Pets and children on the other hand don't look at you with judgement, they simply live in a current state of being, without future thought. When we look at a child or an animal, we become comforted. When a child or animal looks at you, you never feel judged. This is because without knowing it, we feel the power of living and return to the eternal "now," or in a present state of mind. This is the secret to letting go of ego, and simply living without stress.

Once we consciously see ourselves in the things we do and realize that we are all ego-driven we can take the first steps in letting false "self" fall away. This can be difficult to do because the world is living in the shadow of the false self. It's something the entire world does.

Compare how it feels to be around a child or animal versus being around an officer of the law. Many people generally dislike police, because they feel less human around them. Police take on the ego-ic label of officer, and disconnect with people and treat them all the same. As a matter of survival in their jobs, they judge and interact with people on a different level.

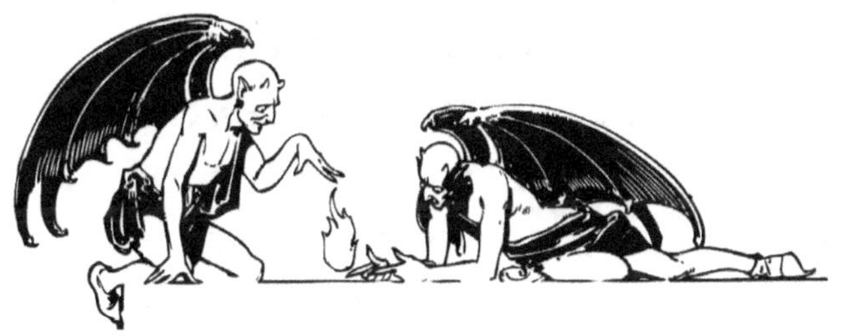

But then sometimes this ego role continues into off-work life. This can happen to any human being. Their label of what they do, becomes who they are, and they are no longer a person, but a constant state of mind. Thus, the goal is to let go of that ego or self-definition, and not let ourselves get taken over.

If we could look without judgment or the ego, we would see the world in a different state all together. We would have patience and less stress. We would know that everything happens for a reason. Rather than getting pissed off that we are in traffic, we would realize that there is nothing we can do about it. We would learn to be grateful and use it as an opportunity to dwell on situations that might arise later in the day.

We can find good in all things, but we choose to dwell on the negative.

The body, being the most primordial (primitive) or basic, is the first thing that one needs to perfect. If the body does not work as the mind wants it to, how then can it function properly as a guide for the mind? Our bodies are the living force that Mother Earth gave us to carry on her will. Our mind is what she gave us to perceive what she has given us, so that we can find love and joy in all things. From the simple smell of flowers, to the beautiful sights of the mountains and rainbows.

But because of the ego and self-rationalization, we not only label ourselves but tell ourselves that we are either not good enough or that we don't deserve the joy life can bring. Like crabs in a bucket when one tried to crawl out, another will pull it back down, making it impossible for anyone to reach the top.

Our society uses guilt to make others feel badly as a form of control. An example of this would be in a relationship, when someone says "If you love me, you would already know what I want, and then do it." Even if they do not say it out loud they still hold that consciousness within. It's how you dominate culture. Oppress someone with a guilt trip.

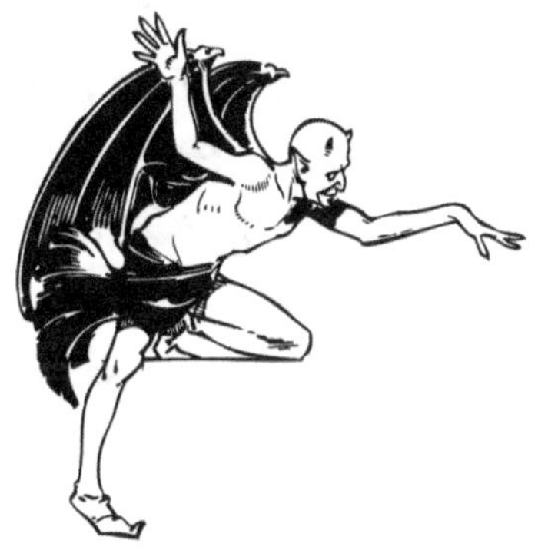

The needs of our ego envelop us as people and even our desires. Sometimes the desire to win, makes it so that we never do. The desire to win is an ego-driven emotion. Yet the state of living in the "present" is not thinking to win. It is thinking… just play the game!

This is what separates the best athletes in the world from others. Do you think that if Tiger Woods didn't have his mind fully in the game, in the "present state" that he could even play as good as he does? There is no way that if he was thinking, "This putt is worth one million dollars," he would ever make it, because the stress of that putt would hinder his game. Rather, he is in the state of what athletes call "the zone." This makes him focus on the task at hand rather than future. He is fully in the present game.

We often times look towards others for our own happiness when it's a selfish egotistical whim. Why would we need anything from without, if we were fully in the moment. The dis-ease of the body, and/or not feeling at home in our body can add to our ego construction. The ego can exist to help us out of pain. Creating a life of Dominant Health can help to remove pain, and thus help to eradicate the ego.

So the object of this game is to release the ego, come back to the present moment, and come back to our God-given nature. I invite you to become in tune with people and things around you, to become more open to seeing life as it is, and not how you might 'project' it to be. It is in this way we are able to step back and see ourselves without judgment and work to better ourselves and humanity.

Raw Matt

FUNDAMENTALS

"It always seems to me that man was not born to be a carnivore."

Albert Einstein

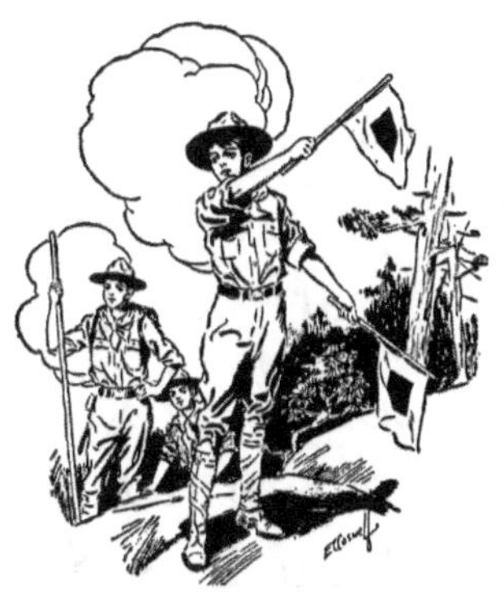

WELCOME

If you were to sit down just a half an hour with a doctor to gather information, they would charge you an arm and a leg, sometimes quite literally! Plus, the information they give you is very often biased by their pharmaceutical training.

Keep in mind that this book is NOT medical advice. This is a gathering of information I have collected from years of reading and research. I have no medical degree, so I have kept much of this information to myself, as I would find myself in jail faster than I could sneeze for practicing without a license.

But God spoke to me and said I must share the Good News that I have found. So as you read this – realize it is just coming from a layperson who has done lots of reading, has an immense passion, and is doing a very long book report! Personally it benefits me nothing to write this, other than to listen to God's call. So I feel that this is information is something we all yearn for.

You are going to come across some subjects in this book that are not normally talked about or discussed, such as physical immortality, effective anti-aging, breatharianism, and non-placebo cleanses. The reason for this is because I have not been swayed or influenced by any company, pharmaceutical industry, product line, or political agenda. You can go buy tons of diet books, exercise books, and raw food guides with ulterior motives, but why bother? I've already read most of them, digested, deciphered, and distilled them to save you major time and effort experimenting and buying all sorts of foods, gadgets & supplements.

If you knew someone in your family was sick or dying, you would not hesitate for a second to give them all your time & knowledge to help them get better. I believe that we are all of the same blood, and this makes us family. All things in life should appeal to reason. When it takes a guru to tell you how to simply live, maybe you should just put past beliefs behind you and live simply, and all will fall into place. So please enjoy this book and be abundantly healthy.

Health is Wealth

There is not a person alive that would choose their wealth over health. Doctor's offices are full of rich and poor people. Ask any terminally ill patient the simple question, "Would you give me all the money you own to rid yourself of this affliction?" You would eagerly hear, "Absolutely!"

The title of this book, Dominant Health is what I want you to feel in abundance. We should never need to rely on someone else when it comes to our own well-being. All the answers are out there and ready for you to learn. Yet in today's culture we are reliant on everyone and everything except ourselves. Ask yourself this, "If you lost everything tomorrow, society collapses, the stock market crashes, what would you do to stay alive?" Our Modern society has lost our ability to sustain ourselves on the land. Sadly I believe we have lost the connection to Mother Earth herself as well.

I wrote this book to give you logical, easy to read information. I have included important lessons that you will want share with others. We have been told countless lies about what we should eat and how we should feel as we age. It is time someone unveils these lie for what their worth and expose ancient hidden truths.

We can fix disease & sickness naturally.

How We Were Designed

I believe that God created us. It is also fine to say we have evolved. To me that's just adaptation and part of God's original creation. Adaptation, however, is not proof of evolution. I don't think we came from moneys.

I actually believe we were fruitarian by design, i.e. meant to live off nothing but fruit and some seeds and herbs. This is what I personally have lived on for years and feel absolutely perfect! But regardless what I believe, there are many scientific facts that confirm my beliefs, including.

- A carnivore has a very short intestinal track that is designed for processing heavy amounts of protein and expelling it before it can begin to putrefy in the body. Our intestinal tract, however, is longer and our hydrochloric acid (stomach acid) is weaker. Unusually high amounts of hydrochloric acid are required by our stomach to digest the proteins found in meat. The digested flesh starts rotting as it makes its way through the longer fruitarian intestinal tract and into the small intestine where nutrients are absorbed. Seeing as it takes up to 48 hours for meat to pass through our bodies, this means that the rotting meat has been releasing harmful bacteria and toxins into our intestines and bloodstream.

- The intestinal track of human closely resembles all fruit eating animals, not herbivores. Herbivores have a lot less stomach acid, much longer intestinal track and often times more stomachs than one. Herbivore primates still have a working appendix. In humans it is vestigial. It has lost its primary function. Every other herbivore in the world uses the appendix to break down plant cellulose. In humans this organ lost that ability and now just stores friendly bacteria (flora). This is why many people get that organ removed without any health problems later in life.

- We have the teeth of a Frugivore, having not jaws that grind side to side like a cow or other plant eating animals, nor do we have a mouth full of sharp canines designed for tearing flesh and meat apart.

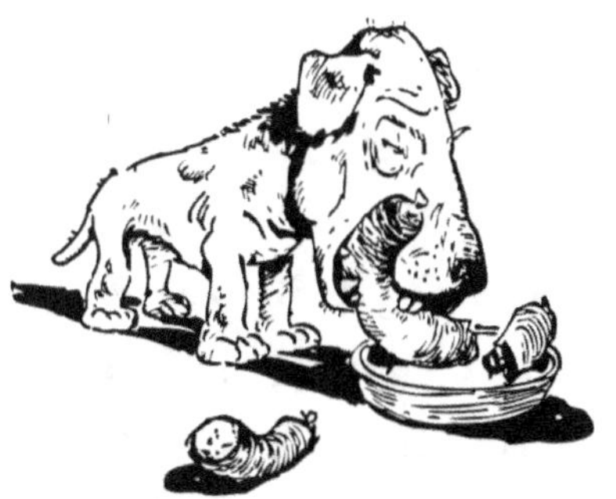

Symbiosis

The Bible says, "Where there is life there is blood." That is the reason we can distinguish what true life is, because it has blood in its veins. So when carnivores make comparisons to killing plant life as akin to killing animal life, there simply is no comparison.

Our blood is made by the nutrients we consume, and our thoughts affect our bodies. Everything works in a symbiotic relationship. I believe that health is not just want we eat, but how we think, the relationships we have with others, spiritual outlook on life and the friends we have. It is body, mind and spirit. All three are a combination of overall health and well-being.

If you have been eating a truly healthy clean living foods diet, then disease can have no hold on you. When we eat incorrectly and become lazy or stagnant then disease is like a moving locomotive in your body. Once that train has momentum, no matter how strong you are, there is no possible way you would stand a chance stopping it. But if you are healthy and moving, disease has no chance of stopping you!

Everything in life is a symbiotic relationship. Just as everything inside our bodies is regulated by communication, the same is true on Earth. The Moon and Earth need each other and without a seemingly unimportant planet like Mars or Venus, Earth would spiral out of control. The Moon acts as a shield to block meteoroids. It controls the axis of the earth, our tides and even plant growth. As herbalists & wine growers know, they harvest grapes on full moon nights.

Without proper sleep, sun light, relaxation, removal of stress, finding our purpose in life, and control of our impulses like emotion, appetite and thought, we are at disharmony. All things are a factor to our health and well being, not just things we ingest.

Philosophic Symbiosis

Deep down on microscopic level we all are exactly the same. For instance it is impossible to tell a person's race looking at DNA. We must take this into consideration when we start looking our own reality.

I find that unless we look into ourselves and see ourselves for who we truly are, we cannot work out our flaws and become better individuals. Most of us are too busy judging others, getting angry, resentful and regretful about the past. We tell ourselves that we have very little time, yet we forget to focus on the things right in front of us and take these blessings for granted.

Take a moment to look at your hand, move all your fingers and think about this for just a moment. What would you give to just be able to do that simple motion if you were born with a deformity? We take such simple things for granted: being able to see, or hear; things that unfortunately many people cannot do.

So rather than dwell on any negative things in life, look at all the positive things. All the negative falls away when you realize how truly blessed you are.

*"Finally, brethren, whatsoever things
are true, honest, just, pure, lovely,
whatsoever things are of good report;
if there be any virtue, and if there worthy
of praise, think on these things."*

Philippians 4:8

How we choose to spend our money is probably the biggest impact we have in this world. We vote with our dollars, we can make a change.

- We vote for the kinds of companies we want to flourish.

- We vote for the kinds of restaurants we wish there were more of.

- We vote for the kinds of shelter we want to see built.

- And we vote by spending our money on organic produce that promotes a sustainable future for many generations to come.

We want to stop consuming things that deplete our top soil such as grains, corn, wheat, rice. These foods are not only unhealthy for our regular consumption, but they cause topsoil erosion. Most of the minerals are not in our soil anymore and today, most of our land cannot even grow trees and we need to plant more trees! Water cannot permeate our soil and things will no longer grow in what was once fertile ground.

Becoming conscious about our foods is the biggest step we can take in our life.

We need to learn how to promote a substantial future for generations to come. Things like dairy and meat consumption are nothing but pollution and rape of our land. It takes over a thousand gallons of water to feed just one cow, and that cow creates huge amounts of waste. This waste in turns creates greenhouse toxins in the environment more than ANY car could. Eighty percent or more of our grains, such as rice, wheat and corn, go to feed cows to feed us. This mindless insane circle of consumption does nothing to promote a sustainable future.

Consider for a moment, that eating out is an activity Americans do on a daily basis.

Now consider that what one single person eats not only directly affects their health, but also the economy, land and resources of the entire planet. As people lose consideration for these things, we eat without consciousness. We are a generation that can have by far, the most impact on this world than any generation before us through our personal actions.

Enzymes

One of the premises of the Raw Food diet and the main consideration of the Raw or Live or Living Food are to maintain the enzymes in your body.

Plant-based digestive enzymes are wonderful to add to any fast, cleanse or daily diet regimen. Enzymes however should be based more on your own special diet, such as whether or not your diet is protein based (meat, legumes eggs, dairy etc.) Carbohydrate based (starchy bread, potatoes, pasta, etc.), or high fat (nuts, oils, seeds etc.).

Let's say you fit into the first category and you consume a high protein diet. Well protein is one of the hardest types of food for the digestive system and usually takes many hours for the body to break down protein into single chain amino acids for assimilation. Therefore you would benefit from an enzyme blend with high amounts of the enzyme named protease. Also a very powerful enzyme for protein is found in papaya and its name is papain. And pineapple enzyme named bromelain really helps in the digestion of protein.

If your diet is more starch based (like mine was before going raw), look for an enzyme blend with the most powerful constituent being lipase. This enzyme is wonderful for its ability to break down starch.

Accumulated starch in the body is one of the biggest problems in America, with the average American carrying an average of 2000-3000 stones in their gallbladder. Gallbladder removal is the number one surgical procedure done in America today, and this is due to our starch-aholic society. Like most people, I love starchy foods and miss pasta the most, but if you continue to consume starchy foods, really consider enzyme therapy for internal health.

When you are a raw foodist most likely your diet consists of high concentrations of fats in your diet. Most raw vegans I personally know are following a regimen with their food pyramid being fat as a base because of their high intake of nuts and seeds as they bypass grains, legumes and dairy. High fat diets are pretty taxing on the body also, and most raw vegans consume high amounts of cocoa, nuts butters, nut milks, raw (un-blanched) nuts and seeds, cereals (nut based) trail mix, & snacks. The enzyme needed predominantly for a raw foodist would then be amylase. As its ability to break down fats and make them more soluble for the body is astounding.

Other amazing enzymes are such proteolytic enzymes such as serratipeptidase (aka serrapeptase). This enzyme is used in other countries other than America to help with inflammation, circulation, cardiovascular support, carpal tunnel, infections, atherosclerosis, sinusitis and bronchitis.

Not much in America has been done to study serratiopeptidase, which is sad. But research I have done shows it acts upon inflammation by thinning the fluids in the body that collect around injured areas and increases fluid drainage. This also enhances tissue repair and reduces pain. Pain is also reduced by the protein enzyme's ability to block amines. Serratiopeptidase also has the unique ability to dissolve the dead and damaged tissue that is a by-product of the healing response without harming living tissue. It is used in this way by the silkworm to digest a hole in the dead tissue of the cocoon so the silkworm can emerge.

Let's not forget about metabolic enzymes, as we have just been mentioning digestive. We could not even consider life without such enzymes as SOD, catalyze & glutathione peroxidase. Every reaction in the body takes place because of these enzymes, from blinking your eyes, flexing your muscles to breathing, all are metabolic reactions created by enzymes.

So no matter what your diet is, remember the enzymes.

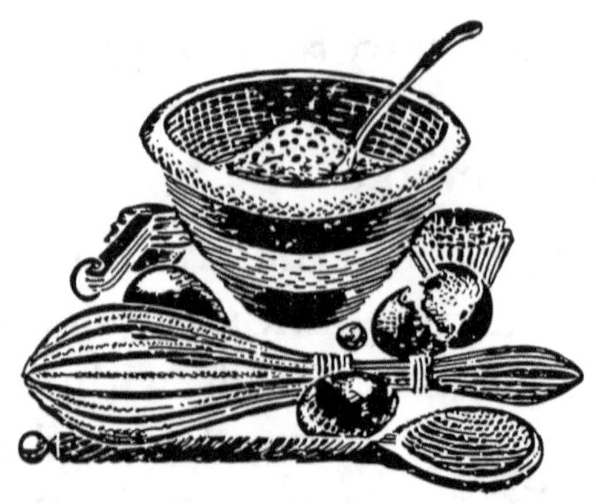

MY BASIC DIETARY RULES

I tend to be very strict with my diet. I never consume breakfast as I stopped doing that years ago. I only eat when the sun is at its highest in the sky and my foods are simple. I consume unheated honey that I harvest myself and water that is from a spring source. I still cleanse and liver flush because I was a starch-oholic and carb-oholic. I am pretty clean now and will continue with my caloric restriction practice and will keep you all posted.

- Skip breakfast, as the word drives from breaking your fast it should only consist of water or a juice for re-hydration from eight hours of sleep (fasting).

- Upon consumption of food always eat sugar first, as sugar digest much faster than protein, and keeps insulin response at bay.

- Keep foods simple, mixing tons of foods together creates havoc in the system and over burdens the body needlessly.

- Never eat till fullness, as this creates mucus formation at a high rate in the body.

- Never eat right before bed, keep solid meals three to four hours before sleep. If you must eat later at night, consume only blended meals or juice two hours before sleep.

- If you have trouble putting on weight stay away from cold drinks as this burns more calories.

- If keeping weight off is an issue, keep metabolism up by using lots of spices, and eat small meals throughout the day. Keep larger meals more spread apart.

Chew Chew Chew

Chewing food is of paramount importance. Our salivary glands secrete lysozyme which kills bacteria. Our saliva also secretes ptyalin that's a type of digestive enzyme, amylase, which digests starch into small segments of multiple and singular soluble sugars. The more starch we consume the more our bodies produce this enzyme, which is amazing! But all this happens ONLY if we chew our food. Otherwise, it puts a strain on our whole digestive system.

Think about a child for a second. Would you give a baby or very young child a piece of meat for nutrition? Of course not. We know that this kind of food is not a good diet. Upon giving a child a piece of meat, they chew and chew because the body knows that this substance cannot be digested properly, and is trying to make up for it in saliva. If a child should not it eat it, then why is it ok for you? Does it not make since to think of nutrition in the same regards? The only thing that happens is we get a stronger immune system that can deal with pathogens much better than a child. This does not mean that the body itself can acquire nutrients from foods any differently than a baby.

Breatharians

On the flip side of chewing – there is breatharianism. I think it's incredibly difficult to go without food or drink indefinitely. I have tried on a few separate occasions. Basically it is simply extreme fasting. I went for four months on just water, and spirulina on every Saturday (Sabbath). My weight dropped from 135 to 115 pounds.

Some people might ask, "What is the difference between breatharianism and starvation?"

Both include not eating. A breatharian may physically stop eating, but it is vastly different. We find nutrients elsewhere. This is why it's impossible to become a breatharian if you are not searching spiritually.

Becoming a breatharian is more than a dietary step but it is also a spiritual one. It consists of putting your faith in Mother Earth knowing that no matter where you are, she will provide for you what you need. Even the poorest places on Earth still can find food in nature. It is about our outlook on food and how we rationalize what "food" really is. I never look at a dog, turkey, pig chicken or cow and think "food". Rather I see fruits, honey and the grass I walk on as super powerful nourishing foods.

Unfortunately most people are not told that this is nourishment, and spend their entire lives sitting on grass while they starve to death.

Most children in foreign countries do not die from starvation. Starvation would mean that they died from no sustenance or nutrients. However these children actually do not die from malnutrition, rather 25% die from a parasitic organism and the rest from a disease. When these children do eat they usually consume cooked white rice or wheat which sets in inflammation (due to indigestible proteins) of the mucus membranes causing a form of Celiac disease.

These starchy foods wreak havoc on the system. They create an acid environment and great hunger and even leaky gut syndrome. It is not the lack of food that causes deficiencies, rather it's what a person has consumed that started disease of the blood. Often these kids have died supposedly of starvation, yet found with rice in their system at time of death. This should tell you something!

I advise anyone who wants to consider being a breatharian to listen to your body and spirit, rather than people who are not living a disease-free thriving life.

Other Essential Ingredients for Breatharians

Water and Mercury are the only two primary liquids found on Earth (aside from lava, a plasma) that are separate from plants and bloods, so we must take that into consideration when looking at drinks to buy and consume. We are literally "liquid" organisms: our bodies contain 55% up to 70% depending on your age, sex and weight. We need to drink water. Water should be the main source of liquid in our diet. Ultimately it makes sense to advance towards a liquid only diet.

Minerals, enzymes, water, fats and salts are what we are made of. They are all found in our cells without need from an outside source if our intestinal flora is in balance. But we do loose some of these things through physical activities, like working out and we need to replenish them.

A small amount of Celtic sea salt in water is not only nice, but it helps us replenish necessary minerals. Plants and seaweeds are also an optimal source for replenishing minerals. Sprouted and ground seeds are your best source for fats and are easily obtainable. These things even in small amounts can keep you far from deficient even when practicing caloric restriction or liquid fasting.

If you give up food without proper background and motivation, don't plan on feeling healthy after a few days. Rather take gradual steps to your goal, starting with cleanses (colon, liver, gall bladder, kidney) fasts (weekly, weekend & new moon). Then progress to a liquids-only regimen. Only then, can you consider stopping everything safely and pursuing breatharianism.

Ultimately, I believe we were created to be able to consume food. The fact that we have teeth is a pretty good testament to this. But we also have the ability to derive much of our nutrients through sunlight, water and breathing as sources of nutrients. Take away any of those three and we lose vitality rather quickly! The positive side of this story is that hunger or starvation, sickness and disease is often a driving force for many people to become seekers of the true meaning of life, and thus seek the true meaning of life and God.

ELEMENTAL NUTRITION

*"If the bee disappears
from the surface of the earth,
man would have
no more than four years to live."*

Albert Einstein

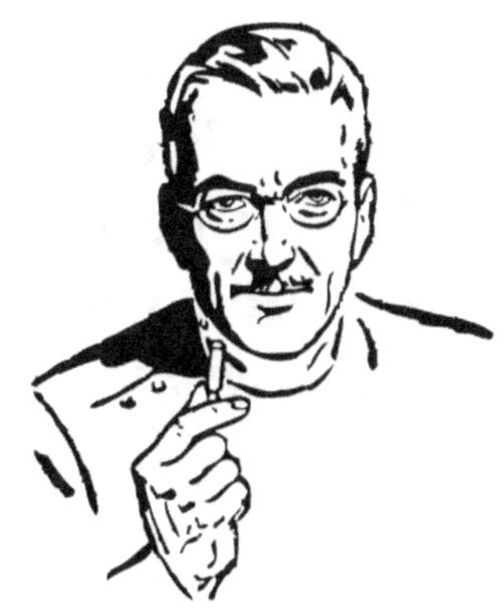

WHY ALTERNATIVE MEDICINE?

Ever wonder why so many people are interested in alternative medicine?

Consider these quotes:

"Over a million patients are injured in hospitals each year, and approximately 180,000 die annually as a result of these injuries. Therefore, the iatrogenic injury rate dwarfs the annual automobile accident mortality of 45,000 and accounts for more deaths than all other accidents combined."

Journal of the American Medical Association

*"150,000 to 300,000 Americans
are injured or killed each year
because of medical negligence
(mistreated diseases, surgeries, drug
reactions, mis-prescribed drugs)."*

Wall Street Journal

*"Iatrogenic diseases, generally defined
as diseases that result from a physician's
action or in response to a drug,
are believed to be a major problem in terms
of morbidity and hospital expense."*

Journal of the American Medical Association

*"Errors in judgment or technique concerning
either the anesthesia or the surgery,
or a combination of the two,
contribute to close to 50% of the mortality
in the operating room."*

Dr. James Mannis,
"Cheating Fate,"
Health

*"Current research suggests that
36% of physician visits are unnecessary;
36% of hospital admissions are caused by
side effects from other medical treatments;
53% of surgeries are unnecessary;
and half of all time spent in hospitals
isn't medically indicated."*

Let's Live

*"Each year, nearly 2 million people in the
United States come down with an infection
in the hospital they didn't have when they
entered; more than 80,000 of these die."*

Let's Live

*"Chemotherapy and radiation
can increase the risk of developing a second
cancer by up to 100 times,
according to Dr. Samuel S. Epstein."*

Congressional Record

*"Stanford University doctors
compared the effects of chemotherapy
to doing nothing in patients with slow
growing tumors of the lymph nodes.
The patients whose treatment was deferred
for years did just as well as patients who
immediately received expensive and
unpleasant chemotherapy.
Nineteen of the 83 (or 23%) experienced
spontaneous remission lasting four months
to six years.*

*A review of the study in the New England
Journal of Medicine concluded, 'deferring
treatment… may allow for spontaneous
regression of the disease.'"*

"Cheating Fate"
Health

*"Of every 1000 American women
getting mammograms each year
between the ages of 40 and 50, 345
will receive false positive results, often
with unnecessary intervention as the result."*

New England Journal of Medicine

*"Harvard researchers
studied hospital records from the state
of New York over a one year period.
They estimated that more than 13,000
New Yorkers were killed
and 2500 were permanently disabled
due to medical care.
More than 51% were blamed
on medical negligence."*

New England Journal of Medicine

*"During 1983-1992,
between 90,000 and 110,000 Americans died
from reactions to prescription drugs,
320 from over the counter drugs,
and 3 from all dietary supplements
combined,
including contaminated L-tryptophan,
and zero from herbs."*

American Association of Poison Control
Centers, FDA, AAPCC, USDA, JAMA,
New England Journal of Medicine.

"44,000 to 98,000 Americans die each year not from the medical conditions they checked in with, but from preventable medical errors.

Two months after a double bypass heart operation that was supposed to save his life, comedian and former Saturday Night Live cast member Dana Carvey got some disheartening news: the cardiac surgeon had bypassed the wrong artery."

fda.gov/fdac/features/2000/500_err.html

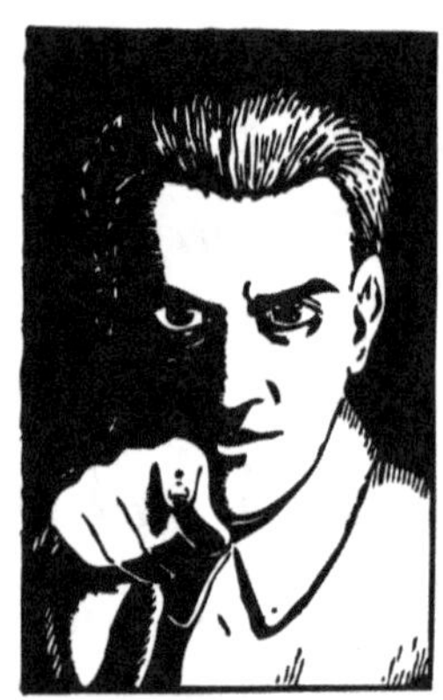

Are you convinced yet, that 'alternative medicine' might be a good alternative?

Medication Errors

The American Hospital Association lists these as some common types of medication errors:

- Incomplete patient information (not knowing about patients' allergies, other medicines they are taking, previous diagnoses, and lab results, for example)

- Unavailable drug information (such as lack of up-to-date warnings)

- Miscommunication of drug orders, which can involve poor handwriting, confusion between drugs with similar names, misuse of zeroes and decimal points, confusion of metric and other dosing units, and inappropriate abbreviations

- Lack of appropriate labeling as a drug is prepared and repackaged into smaller units

- Environmental factors, such as lighting, heat, noise, and interruptions, which can distract health professionals from their medical tasks.

Numerous drugs approved since 1993 have been withdrawn after reports of death and severe side effects such as: Lotronex, Redux,

Raxar, Posicor, Duract, Rezulin, and Propulsid. I have a lot to write about drugs but this article pretty much explains it all. "Deadly Mix at the FDA" by David William from the Los Angeles Times. You should be able to read it online and it present the facts on why you should Western Medical pharmaceuticals, unless it is an emergency. David Willman's special report won a Pulitzer Prize for investigative reporting. Thank you David Willman!

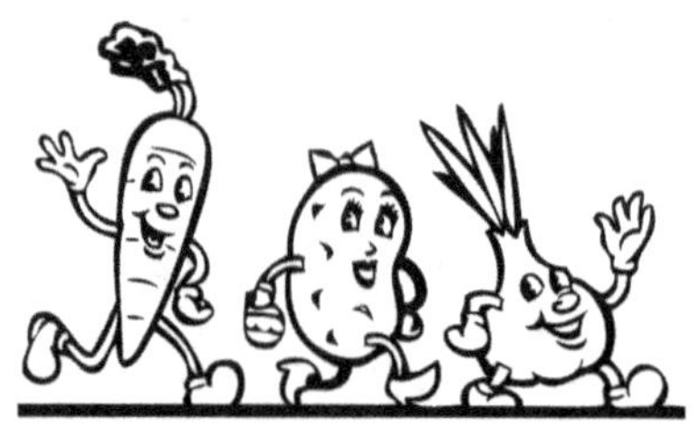

What to Eat?

Organic Produce!

The suffix "cide" comes from Latin and means to kill, killer; murder, to cause death, slayer. Our pesti(cide), herbi(cide), fungi(cide), insecti(cide) laden produce is contaminating our water, land, environment and our bodies. Only obtain Organic produce, grown without the use of these death-causing chemicals.

The majority of the following data comes from the U.S. Government agencies and their respective reports. Data was also assembled in July 2005 by Craig Minowa Environmental Scientist, for the Organic Consumer Association. All sources of this data can be found at www.organicconsumer.org along with more information...

The US Soil Conservation Service estimates that more than three billion tons of topsoil erodes from US croplands each year. They state that "soil is eroding seven times faster than it is being built up naturally." They agree that "American farms are now suffering from the worst soil erosion in history" which can lead to desertification and dust bowls. Organic farming is fundamentally about nourishing & building up healthy, nutrient rich topsoil.

And here are some more U.S. Government facts. According to the Environmental Protection Agency (EPA) and the National Academy of Sciences, noxious chemicals are up to ten times more toxic to children than adults. This is due to the fact that children take in more toxic chemicals relative to body weight than adults. They have developing organ systems that are more vulnerable and less able to detoxify toxic chemicals.

- According to EPA's Guidelines for Carcinogen Risk Assessment, "Children receive 50% of their lifetime cancer risks in the first two years of life."

- According to the Food and Drug Administration, half of produce currently tested in grocery stores contains measurable residues of pesticides.

- Laboratory tests of eight baby foods reveal the presence of sixteen pesticides, including three carcinogens.

- In blood samples of children age two to four, concentrations of pesticide residues are six times higher in children eating conventionally farmed fruits and vegetables compared to those eating organic.

- Currently over, 400 chemicals can be regularly used in conventional farming as biocides to kill weeds and insects. For example, apples can be sprayed up to sixteen times with thirty six different pesticides. None of these chemicals are present in organic foods.

- Over 300 synthetic food additives are allowed by the FDA in conventional foods. None of these are allowed in foods USDA certified organic

The U.S. Department of Agriculture strictly prohibits mixing different types of pesticides for disposal, due to the well-known process of the individual chemicals combining into a new highly toxic chemical compounds. However, there are no regulations regarding pesticide mixtures on a consumer product level, even though, in a similar manner, those same individual pesticide residues interact and mix together into new chemical compounds when conventional multiple ingredients products are made. 62% of food products tested contain a measurable mixture of residues of at least three different pesticides.

Exposure to Organophosphate Pesticides (OP) is linked to hyperactivity, behavior disorders, learning disabilities, developmental delays and motor dysfunction. OPs account for half of the insecticides used in the US. According to the U.S. Department of Health And Human Services, OPs are now found in the blood of 95% of Americans tested! OP levels are twice as high in the blood samples taken from children than in adults. The U.S. Centers for disease Control reports that one of the main sources of pesticide exposure for the U.S. Children comes from the food they eat.

Perchlorate is well known as a major component in rocket fuel. It is also used as a pesticide. In sufficient amounts it disrupts the thyroid by inhibiting the uptake of iodide, an essential component of thyroid hormones. Because these hormones direct brain development, health concerns have focused on fetuses and young infants.

So eat Organic!

Genetically Modified Organisms (GMOs)

Today humans cross tomatoes and flounder (a fish!) genes to make the tomato more cold resistant, and corn with snake venom to increase pest resistance. Soy, unless it specifically states it is organic, has been genetically modified and wreaks absolute havoc in our bodies, disrupting hormones and deregulating body systems.

Obviously, there is no thought of health implications. Rather, money is the motivating factor. These unnatural GMOs result in higher profits and cheaper production costs, all at a greater expense to our health. You do not have to participate in this degradation. Remember, you vote with your dollar.

Avoid GMOs easily by looking at the produce sticker. If it starts with a three, avoid it. It is GMO. If the number starts with a four, this means it has been sprayed with numerous chemicals.

Only buy produce with a sticker that starts with the number nine or has been locally grown and promised to be chemical-free. If you are buying packaged ready-to-eat goods, be sure that the label states it contains organic ingredients, or specifically that it contains no GMOs.

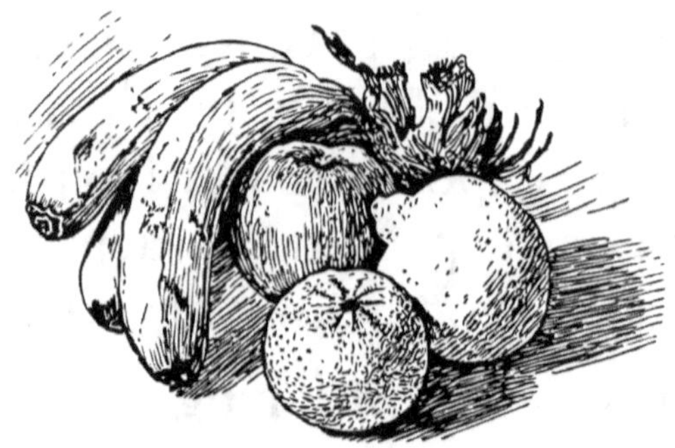

FRUGIVORES

As already mentioned, we are Frugivores!

Try to eat mainly low sugar flowers and fruits like Cauliflower and Cucumber, And take into consideration that each person has different metabolism, health conditions, diseases (fungus, yeasts, etc..), but in general we all work the best on what nature has given us as food. And what nature supplies us is the highest optimal nourishment for our bodies.

Foods grown nowadays are depleted of many minerals, but this does not mean that they are all bad, just less nutritious. Consider for a moment that if you were stranded on a deserted island, would you starve to death if you could not find a restaurant? Odds are some actually would! But in general, no.

Foods that one can forage in the wild are often times a thousand times more nutrient rich than foods grown on a farm. Wild foods have much higher mineral content, higher sulfur content, lower sodium to potassium ratio, and more raw life force than anything that's been grown for mass production. And heirloom varieties of fruits and vegetables are always preferred when you must buy commercial produce. Heirloom plants are closer to their original traits through open pollination, and not commonly found in modern large-scale agriculture. Whereas most commercial produce has been propagated through the centuries through grafts and cuttings.

With that in consideration organic, locally grown fresh herbs and fruit are optimal, unless you want to harvest your own foods in the wild. This takes a skilled eyes and time to learn. I advise one when shopping to look for monocot (liliopsida) fruits and stay further away from dicots (magnoliopsida), i.e. fruits such as pineapple, banana & other seedless fruits! Not only do more sugary fruits cause runaway sugars in the body, but they are very weak in comparison to their counterpart, the monocot.

I recommend eating foods like (heirloom) cucumber, olives, cherries, apricots, peaches, coconuts, cantaloupe, cauliflower, berries (strawberry, cranberry, blueberry, raspberry, camu camu, goji, blackberries, Incan, mulberries, acai, etc...) mangostean, figs, papaya, nectarines, citrus (orange, tangerine, lemon, grapefruit, lime etc...), plums, dates (heirloom only), grapes, honeydew, pumpkin, avocados (high omega 6s), apple (careful most have fungus – see my later notes), pears (although hard on intestines), and finally bee products which are derived from the pollen of fruits: honey, pollen, royal jelly.

Eat Raw

Everything I speak of consuming has natural enzymes, so I do not advise cooking many foods. Naturally, I believe that steaming vegetables and greens, that are high in starch or cellulose, such as such as broccoli, kale, cabbage, and cauliflower. If you really want to eat these foods, cooking these foods is alright, because we were really not designed to eat them in the first place, and this helps to eliminate the hard-to-digest elements. Juicing, blending, and fermenting are also great ways to assimilate nutrients.

I advocate a little juicing and lots of blending and making soups out of foods like cabbage, broccoli, cilantro, watercress, radish, kale, chard greens, chlorella, collard greens, dandelions, edible flowers, fermented veggies, kohlrabi, lettuce, mushrooms, mustard greens, onions, parsnips (high glycemic and not recommended), peppers, tomatoes, spinach, eggplant (nightshade's be careful), rutabaga (buckwheat), sea veggies (dulse, kelp, nori, etc...), spirulina, sprouts, wheat grass, wild greens, parsley, celery, ginger, garlic, and other vegetables.

Blended foods not only make for much better assimilation, it can make the food more interesting as opposed to just making a massive salad.

Nuts and Seeds

Nuts and seeds are all harder on the digestive track because as nuts from trees they usually contain enzyme inhibitors. These anti-nutrients are the plants built-in protective resource enabling them to sprout out of season. For the human body to take most nutritional value from nuts and seeds we must go about sprouting, blending and perhaps culturing & chewing them well for full absorption.

Seeds in nature were designed to pass through the digestive track, eliminated in the stool, and start the process of growing into another tree. The nuts and seeds that are the best are hemp seeds, pine nuts (a goitrogen – avoid if you have hypothyroidism), pumpkin seeds, Brazil nuts, walnuts, pecans, flax (be sure to soak and strain before consumption as it contains hydrogen cyanide), chia and sunflower seeds, macadamias and almonds.

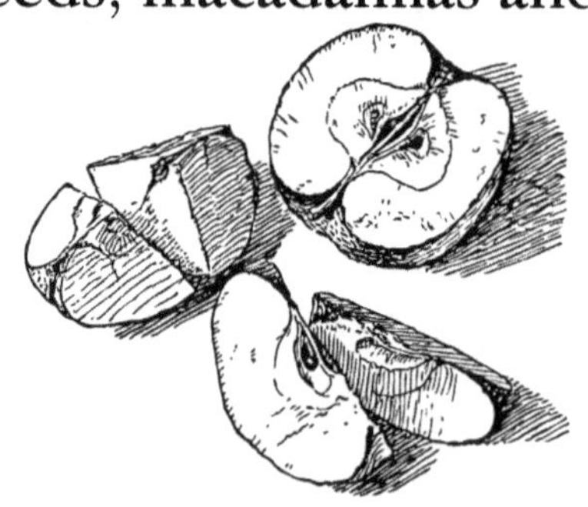

Apples

Foods like apples & pears contain high amounts of fungus. Over the years they have been genetically modified and made weak, because they cannot defend themselves like they normally would in nature. Many commercially bred plants share this characteristic. In nature most things have a bitter taste. In order to survive, a plant will make alkaloids so it's less attractive to an animals taste its buds. It also gives it a lot more ability to resist fungus and molds.

The common apple and pear contain rotting fungi, penicillin expansum and monilinia fructigena. This is a new concern as the fungus and parasites live just under the skin and has the appearance of an innocuous bruise or soft spot. When obtaining a fresh apple or pear immediately refrigerate and before consumption peal it. Most apples are shipped fresh but sit on shelves at room temperature, making them ripen too fast. Try to obtain the freshest apples possible - the smaller the more flavor, and refrigerate ASAP.

Oxalate Foods

Peanuts are among a small number of foods that contain measurable amounts of oxalates (a form of calcium), naturally-occurring substances found in plants, animals, and human beings. When oxalates become too concentrated in body fluids, they can crystallize and cause health problems in the kidney, gallbladder and other organs. Potassium when taken with magnesium, can help prevent calcium-oxalate kidney stones.

If you are prone to kidney stones, gallbladder issues, or arthritis, the following list may prove helpful to you:

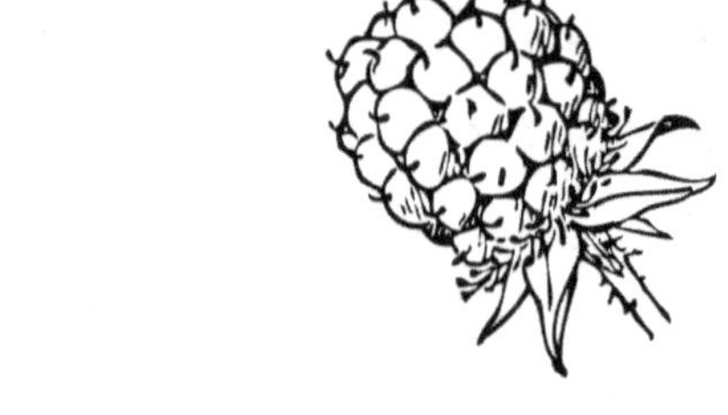

- Avoid fruits high in Oxalates: blueberries, strawberries, currants, lemon, lime, & orange peels, purple grapes, rhubarb, dewberries, figs, gooseberries & kiwi.

- Limit fruits moderate in oxalates: apples, blackberries, raspberries, cranberries, apricots, cherries, grapefruit, green grapes, oranges, peaches, pears, pineapple, plums & prunes.

- Enjoy fruits low in oxalates: avocado, bing cherries, cantaloupe, lemon & lime juice, mango, coconut, honeydew melon, watermelon, nectarines, papaya & raisins.

- Avoid vegetables high in oxalates: beets, celery, collards, dandelion greens, eggplant, escarole, green beans, kale, leeks, okra, parsley, parsnips, peppers green, pokeweed, popcorn, potatoes, sweet potatoes, pumpkin, rhubarb, rutabagas, sorrel, spinach, yellow squash, summer squash, Swiss chard, tomato, turnip greens, watercress, yams.

- Limit vegetable moderate in oxalates: asparagus, artichokes, Brussels sprouts, broccoli, carrots, corn (sweet, white, or yellow), cucumber, garlic, kohlrabi, lettuce, (butter, iceberg), mushrooms, mustard greens, onions, radishes, snow peas, watercress.

- Enjoy vegetables low in oxalates: acorn squash, all sprouts (alfalfa, broccoli etc.), cabbage, cauliflower, peeled cucumber, red pepper, turnips, zucchini squash.

- A diet high on liquids also will help flush the kidneys of many impurities along with high potassium supplementation one can dissolve stones in a few months. Try adding lemon juice to your water daily.

Bananas

So much of today's food is weak due to it being hybrid & genetically altered, especially bananas.

The term anthracnose literally means "black coal" and is used to describe a disease which spreads black spots on leaves or fruits. Anthracnose is common of today's banana, caused by the fungus colletotrichum musae. Because of the genetically weak integrity of modern day bananas, this fruit would not grow at all without intervention from man. If a simple twenty-five mile an hour wind blows into a banana field it gets completely wiped out. We have genetically killed our banana and because of this malcontent I believe our grandkids will not get to taste a banana.

Small, blackish brown & sunken lesions of this disease appear only after the fruit has ripened. But the initial infection actually starts on the green fruits before they are even harvested, when spores of the fungus land on the fruits surface. They germinate and produce a small, local induced infection. This infection however remains hidden and undetected until the fruit ripens and turns yellow. At this stage the fungus resumes its growth in the skin, and eventually the lesions blossom, causing blemishes & soft spots visible to anyone.

All bananas bought today will show this fungus if left to ripen. Most of us see these spots as just age spots and think it's normal. This process of making the fungus spread faster is induced by damage to the skin during shipping and handling. Manufacturing facilities try to prevent this by dipping all bananas in fungicide before shipping. Regardless if organic or not, refrain from bananas if you can.

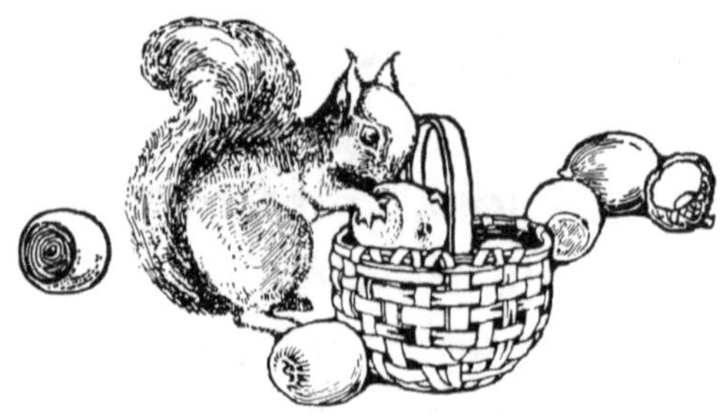

Non-Fruit Foods

Soy and Legumes

Never find legumes as a source of nourishment, as their fungus concentration is simply too high to be nourishment for the human body in the long run. Legumes form as symbiotic relationship with both bacteria in soil and mycorrhizal fungi. Some fungi are parasitic whereas others, like mycorrhizal fungi, take nutrition from plants but give something back in return. Mycorrhizal is a fungus found in soil and needed for plant nourishment, as where the fungus I am speaking of is found on legumes (peanuts, cashews, etc..) This is why peanuts are against the law in most schools now to give to kids. Even being around the vapor can cause death! Almonds now are similar to peanuts, as they also contain higher amounts of aflatoxins (fungi).

Herbs

Without getting into too many specific herbs, I want to touch a little bit on herbalism. One of the long lost natural cures has been sadly overlooked because pharmacology reigns supreme in modern day society.

The multibillion dollar industry makes valid commercial marketing of natural herb remedies almost impossible. This is because patents cannot be put on nature. Only the active ingredients or compounds (plant alkaloids) can be standardized and patented. Although 25% or more of today's medicine comes from plant sources, herbalism is still shunned. A good example is aspirin which is derived from White Willow bark alkaloid. The medicinal content in white willow sitting in health food stores is regulated and WAY under powered so it lacks its full ability to heal.

Gotu Kola

On of my favorite herbs is gotu kola which helps blood travel to the brain, improves brain function, and reduces the stress response. I feel it helps physical strength as well. Unfortunately most the scientific studies done with gotu kola have been on rats so they limited validity for humans. In the only controlled clinical trial on gotu kola and anxiety, published in the Journal of Clinical Psychopharmacology in 2000, scientists gave forty healthy adults either a very high one-time dose of twelve gram dose of gotu kola or a placebo. Then they measured the subjects' startle responses with loud bursts of noise. After sixty minutes, the gotu kola group displayed less than half the startle response of the control group. This is excellent news, as stress is a huge problem and one of the leading root causes of degenerative diseases and death.

Ashwaganda

Adaptogenic herbs like ashwagandha are known for their ability to stimulate Super Oxide Dismutase (SOD). This metabolic enzyme helps to increase the body's immune system and endurance. Ashwagandha can be used by both men and women, Ashwagandha acts to calm the mind and promote sound, restful sleep. Ashwagandha works as an adaptogen, promoting the body's ability to maintain homeostasis and resist stress, anxiety and fatigue. But most people do not know that this herb also promotes dendrite growth in the brain, i.e. the branched projections of neurons that make electrochemical stimulation connections. If taken daily for four months, improvement can be seen in the area of memory. Two studies done in Japan indicate that Ashwagandha also stimulates the growth of axons (connections in the brain). This is significant because the growth of dendrites and axons may compensate for and repair damaged neuronal circuits in the dementia brain or Alzheimer's addled brain.

Ashwagandha antioxidant properties have also been shown to help protect the brain from damage in several other studies, including one in which it was used as a prophylactic against damage caused by stroke. Ashwagandha.net promotes Ashwagandha as a remedy of various health problems, nervous disorders, intestinal infections, and impotency. Above all, it is popularly used by physicians in India as a powerful aphrodisiac.

That's just a few herbs I like, and there are literally thousands of herbs on earth. Herbs have been used all over this planet for medicinal use since the earliest days of man. Even the famous prehistoric caveman drawings in the Lascaux Caves in France depict the use of herbs.

MSM

MSM is promoted as a natural source of sulfur by the supplement and health food industry. The efficacy of MethylSulfonylMethane (MSM) has been questioned. They suggest that people are deficient in sulfur intake, when in fact protein in the diet is usually an abundant source of sulfur. Sulfur is contained in the amino acids methionine and cysteine. I personally love MSM but only consume it during times of injury as MSM is acidic and should not be taken on a continual basis.

Starches

You might wonder what is wrong with starch and that is a good question. Starch is actually not very prevalent in nature but yet found mostly being grown or propagated for human consumption. The whole base of the current food pyramid is basically starch. Most of these starchy foods like potatoes, corn, legumes, rice & wheat all contain indigestible proteins like gliadin & glutenin. These foreign indigestible proteins cause inflammation of the mucus membrane and essentially are the root cause for Celiac Disease.

Starch continually leaves debris behind inside the body that accumulates and wreaks havoc on the system. When it enters the body, starch breaks down into carbonic acid in the blood. Carbonic Acid is a byproduct of Carbon Dioxide and one of the things that is acidifying and changing the pH balance of the ocean as well. Just as the ocean pH is changed, starch acidifies the human body, too. A system that is acid is a whole other topic, but basically, it's not good. Essentially most people walk around in a very acid condition and it is a major factor is disease and illness.

Starch from the Standard American Diet (SAD) also turns into stones in our gallbladder that accumulate over the years. The average American can have well over 1000 of them!

Starch when cooked is even worse. When potatoes are cooked a known carcinogen results that robs the body of zinc. Many kids have acne due to this zinc deficiency. Zinc helps keep sebum (skin oil) sterile. But without it, the fat in the body becomes rancid and contributes to the proliferation of acne bacteria.

So after some good fasting and cleansing, and eating more of a raw living foods diet, there's more work to do to deal with years of starch abuse. The best way to do this is to use herbs and cleanses focused on the liver and gallbladder.

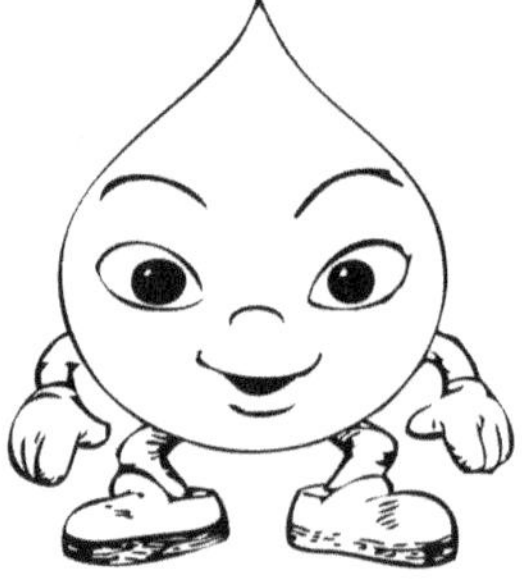

Water

The average system is continuously under bombardment with all the heavy dense dead food we feed it and that stresses the liver greatly. So water is the most important substance you need daily. It should be the most high end item obtainable in your diet.

My personal favorite water is natural spring water from the source, and from a reputable known spring. Nothing is more nutritious and filled with life force than that. Test the water for dissolved solids (make sure the number is lower than 100), and is parasites and bacteria-free, then drink worry free as you are consuming the more pure solution in all of Earth.

If you are absolutely NOT able to obtain your water from a natural spring and you must buy it, then I advise looking for spring water packaged in GLASS, or de-ionized water. Deionization is better than distillation. It gets out all chlorine and fluoride without the mineral leaching effects of distillation.

If you buy your water in plastic, transfer it to glass before refrigeration, as temperature change causes plastic leakage into the water. If you buy distilled, add a small amount of Celtic sea salt to a gallon to add some minerals back in.

Be aware that many companies pump calcium into bottled water to make it more alkaline. Although the liver can process over 3000 pounds of calcium alone in a lifetime and over 80,000 pounds of food (that's over forty tons!) it's best to give it a rest now and then… If you have no other choice, look for distilled because it will not stress the body any more than it has to be. Water without any minerals in it, is very easy on the body.

Alkaline water is not necessary and can actually be harmful. The naturally occurring pH of water is between 7.2 and 7.6, and our own body's pH is also slightly above neutral; around 7.4. Our stomach acid is highly acidic around a pH of 2. Introducing artificially alkaline water is something the body does not want and will work to neutralize or expel as quickly as possible. This is why many people bloat and experience a diuretic affect from drinking watermelon juice a highly alkaline melon. It is best to avoid gimmicky, expensive contraptions like "kangen" water systems and purchase a reliable quality water filter made of high grade carbon. Look for an iodine rating of 1000 or more.

A note of caution: highly alkaline water is toxic to cats. Dogs are a little more adaptable to any water.

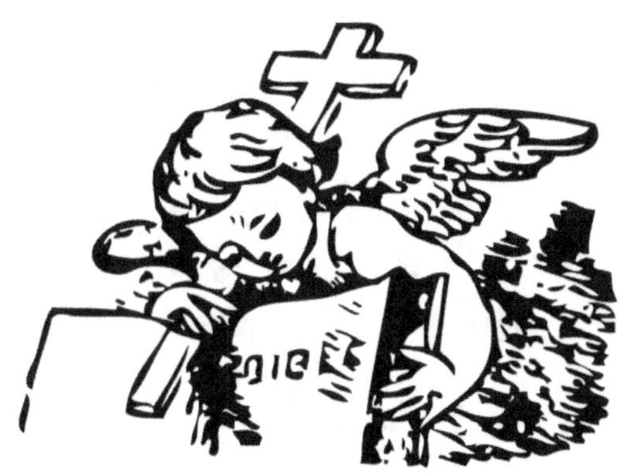

EAT BY INTUITION

You know deep down what your body needs. Sometimes I consume too much honey and my body sends me to a salt craving, then I satisfy that and feel great. Most of us have read how salt is bad for you or sugar in honey is bad. But rather than relying on what you read, try various raw foods yourself, and see how your body feels on each. I suggest that people keep on a low glycemic diet predominantly primarily consisting of fruit. If you work out a lot reach for more greens & nuts, as "green makes clean."

Just listen to your body and it will guide you.

Mother Earth knows what we need, and she provides it for you. Look around at the abundant green color all over the planet and draw your own conclusions what we should be eating. All around us are her precious gifts, grown from her womb and this abundant food is nurturing, not only for us, but the whole planet. It was the way we were meant to eat, the way we were designed.

Eating by Blood Type

The book, <u>Eating for Your Blood Type,</u> shows which foods might aggravate the body if you have a specific blood type. It is based off the lectins in the blood. But as far as the foods that are good for you, the author simply pulls them out of thin air. As far as I'm concerned any author that doesn't mention a single thing about enzymes needs to be overlooked as a nutritionist. Consider looking at foods by how they build healthy blood and you will find that certain foods build good blood in everyone regardless of gender or race or blood type.

All blood is built from the foods we eat and by our spleen & intestinal flora. We are in complete control of how clean our blood is by what we put in our mouths. For instance, chlorophyll builds better blood than anything, and is found in green vegetables. And all the information contained in the rest of this book will be a strong comprehensive guide on how to build the best blood possible – blood that fungus, mold, bacteria, yeast, viruses and parasites cannot live in!

Fats

When people hear the word fat, they get turned off. When in reality fat is a great thing to have in a diet. In fact, a diet void of all fat is actually unhealthy. Natural fats from nuts, seeds & fruits are the best in the world for your health. Your body uses fat, not only as energy, but for many processes of the body, such as helping to balance cholesterol, which in turn helps to regulate hormones.

Although fat content should be on the low end of total consumed calories (about 15-20%), never adhere to a non-fat diet. The Standard American Diet encourages a typical fat content of around 45%! Even raw foodists consume an average of 40% fat due their high intake of nuts, seeds, and their oils and butters. If someone tells you, "Go ahead and eat a jar of almond butter – it's raw so you can't gain weight!" don't believe it for a second. However, the more active you are, the more fats are safely allowed to consume without gaining weight or body fat percentage. Like sugar, fats (especially medium chain triglyceride, or MCTs) are our energy source.

I make use of predominantly olive, acai, chia, coconut and hemp oils. As far as nuts and seeds go, when they are sprouted they become a lot easier to digest. I tend to push people to hemp seeds as they contain no enzyme inhibitors (means no sprouting required) and have great ratio of Omega 3 to 6 fats, and they also contain Omega 9 and 18, with all the essential amino acids and many minerals. However, be sure not to overdue hemp oil, as it is slightly estrogenic and may cause hormonal imbalance.

Grains are not used too often in the raw food world because they are very hard to work with and digest. Modern day agricultural grains contain lots of fungus and are mostly hybridized, making them incredibly difficult to consume and nutritionally weak. Emmer wheat is the original wheat, pre-dating spelt, and contains very low starch. Once sprouted, it has very little starch left. This strong 'father of wheat' is very resistant to fungus, whereas today's hybrids are usually laced with chemicals and prone to fungus, molds and bacteria infections. If you can find Emmer, you can indulge in it in limited quantities. However, I still tend to push people off grains all together.

It is important to take consideration to your ratio of Omega 3 to 6 ratios. We want somewhere around 1 to 5 ratio of Omega 3 to 6. Yet the average human is somewhere around a one to twenty ration with almost no 3s in our diet and tons of Omega 6 fats that are very inflammatory. High amounts of Omega 6 foods often result in skin disorders like acne and eczema. Foods like avocado and olive are higher in Omega 6. Keep spirulina, chia, hemp, coconut and borage as your main source of fats. These bring in anti-inflammatory properties and fats like GLA (Gamma Linolenic Acid) a substance prostaglandins can be made from. Avoid sunflower, safflower, canola, sesame, and peanut oil. These are all inflammatory oils that throw off your body's Omega ratios.

Fish

Do not obtain your fats from fish or fish oils (these are pressed from fish livers, which contain any number of toxins that the liver naturally stores and filters). Continual consumption of fish will always lead to an enzyme deficiency of thiaminase. If you do eat fish, ensure that they are small cold-water fish like salmon or halibut (this translates to lower mercury contamination and a healthier fish), and do not consume more than twelve ounces (about 2-3 servings) in one week.

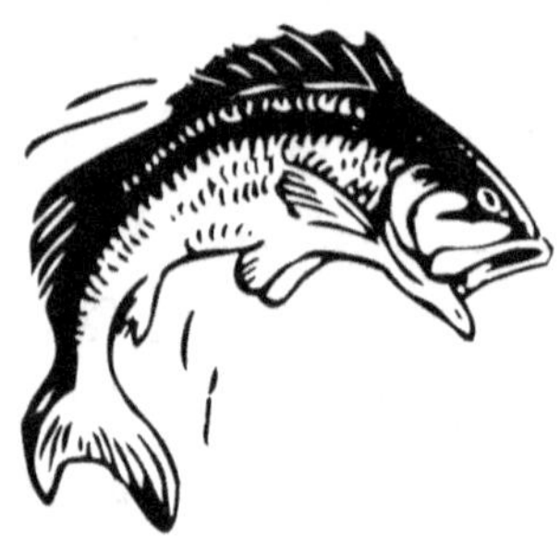

Plant Fats VS. Animal or Fish Fats

Most plant fats are superior to animal fats for several reasons. One is that ALL animal fats increase LDL Cholesterol. Whereas with plant fats one can find an array of health benefits all the way from reducing inflammation to boosting immune system. Sterolins & sterols are fats found only in plants such as seaweed, sprouts, vegetables, fruits, seeds herbs and trees. Plant fats can lower LDL cholesterol levels, increase T-cell function & bring down inflammation. As with many things, moderation is key.

Salt

Since our blood is 0.9% salt and it is continually flowing through our lymphatic system its importance is vital. It is also necessary for the production of hydrochloric acid, the digestive enzyme secreted by the stomach in order to digest protein. It is important for nerves and muscles. When you sweat you can taste the salt coming out of your skin, thus it is very important to replace salt, especially for athletes.

Put a salt block outside and all animals will consume it. Put a calcium block and no animal will even look at it. We should take the animal kingdoms intuitiveness.

An eight-year study of a New York City hypertensive population stratified for sodium intake levels found those on low-salt diets had more than four times as many heart attacks as those on normal-sodium diets. This was the exact opposite of what the "salt hypothesis" would have predicted. Although this bears more investigation, I believe that this is because salt has biological transmutation properties.

Living on a diet low in salt can eventually lead to dehydration. As salt holds water in the body, people can actually dehydrate and die drinking water! Our ancient ancestors knew this, and even nature shows this when we inspect the flora. This is why desert climate plants contain high levels of salt, as this helps the body retain and hydrate the body better.

Sodium relaxes the adrenals and combats chronic fatigue syndrome. Sodium helps the emulsification of fats and oils and along with other minerals promotes cell respiration. Try this little experiment: rub sea salt on kale and watch the plant cellulose break down. The kale leave will almost literally evaporate. Sodium is important for cardiovascular health and buffers shock done to the body similar to glucose. Lastly, I am not a fan of any rock salt, even pink Himalayan crystal salt. Celtic Sea salt is optimal, as bacteria are unable to survive in seawater and the body readily absorbs nutrients in this form.

As a vegetation or vegan, salt is more than important. Lots of meats and blood contain sodium naturally and not consuming these foods, it's important we have some form of salt in the body. Just remember that in order to have optimum sodium intake, it is important to drink water exclusively. Avoid getting sodium from soda, sports drinks, and other beverages, as this will simply dehydrate you. Consuming large quantities of dehydrated foods AND salt on a raw food diet is not the best idea.

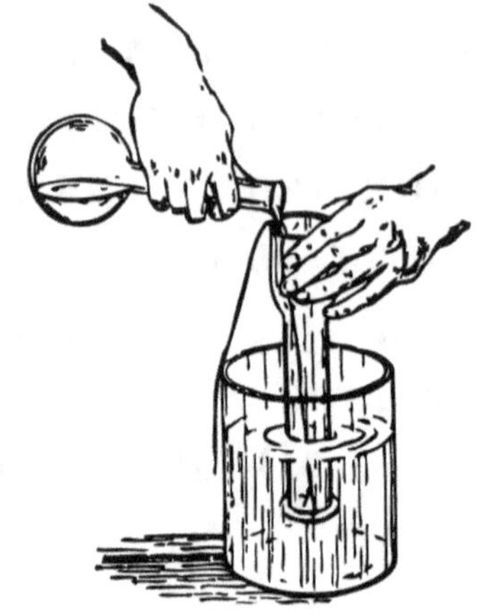

SUPPLEMENTS

Spirulina and B 12

Spirulina is an amazing food source containing all 72 minerals of the body (if grown right) with all the B vitamins including B12. Most people don't know that on the moon they are growing spirulina for its powerful ability to turn sunlight into usable oxygen. This powerful micro algae differs from sun chlorella but is just as powerful in different ways. Sun Chlorella is a genus of single-celled green algae. When it was discovered in the 1940s it was thought to be the answer to world hunger.

Spirulina is a powerful supplement and considered a superfood meaning it's almost able to fly and leap tall buildings. Regardless of this special ability it has a really strong effect on people with weakening bones and also can alkalize a system fast. A two week fast on spirulina and honey can revitalize a person's blood and bones. Honey has the ability to help calcium absorb and Spirulina contains a most usable form of calcium with double the amount of magnesium in perfect proportions.

I personally love spirulina. It is a powerful addition to smoothies, salads and even fruit. It contains healthy fats like gamma-linolenic acid (GLA), alpha-linolenic acid (ALA), linoleic acid (LA), stearidonic acid (SDA), eicosapentaenoic acid (EPA), docosahexaenoic acid (DHA), and arachidonic acid (AA). These are substances not readily found in many other foods, but are very helpful for the human body and brain.

B-12 from spirulina is not utilized by the body as well as one might think. The body actually has a hard time obtaining B-12 from any food. This vitamin is recycled in the body, but as we age it diminishes leaving people with less and less vitality.

B-12 helps the body fight infections, HIV, building of blood cells, CoQ10 energy production, & it also helps lower levels of homocysteine in the blood. Other roles of B12 include proper nervous system development and prevention of infertility in men. Studies also show its ability to improve memory, eye sight and promote heart health. Low amounts of B12 can create a deficiency or absorption problems eventually leading to pernicious anemia, chronic fatigue, weakness, loss of appetite, constipation, poor memory, and depression.

The most common form of B12 on the market is cyanocobalamin. Cyanocobalamin is synthetic and does not occur in nature, and is not used directly in the human body or that of any other animal. But animals and humans can convert it to active forms of the vitamin if the body is healthy.

I tend to push people towards a multi B vitamin complex called NANO B complex. This supplement is scientifically proven to help the body absorb B-12 more then any other supplement or food on the market.

Minerals

I have been asked if mineral supplements, colloidal minerals, Himalayan sea salts are good mineral alternatives? To me, they are absolutely not. Minerals come in different forms and like all nutrients we put into our bodies, it's all about what we can assimilate.

Most mineral supplements are derived from ground up soil, clay, rocks, or even shells. These types of minerals are known as metallic hydrophobic minerals. This literally means they are not water soluble. Unlike minerals you derive from a plant source, these minerals are not utilized by the body and can be a great burden in the long run. The minerals that are the best are sea minerals derived from seaweeds such as kelp, dulse & nori and are even far superior to Celtic sea salt.

Angstrom minerals are smaller than colloidal and even more bio-available. Better, digest your minerals from plants, which derive their minerals from the soil. This is why it's so important to ingest the most mineral rich, soil-grown plants possible and derive mineral supplementation from foods: herbs, flowers, fruit, bee products, vegetables and ocean, not the water you drink, rocks, clay or anything man made. These tend to be inferior in comparison.

Be leery when you hear about super minerals like humic and fulvic acids that claim to turn inorganic minerals already pre-existing in the body into something usable. It's also said fulvic acid helps as a carrier to herbal compounds to help permeate deeply into the tissues of muscle. The form of these acids also hook toxins and escort them out of the body, it's a process known as bio-availability enhancer. The best form to obtain these minerals from is shilijit. I'll let you do your own research on this, but below I'll list what it is and where it's found.

Shilajit

Shilijit is a complex but completely natural black, gummy mixture of minerals with organic and inorganic compounds that is gathered off Himalayan mountain faces. It looks like bat or rodent droppings! It is one of the most important Rasayana tonics in Ayurveda that speeds wound healing. It is the first treatment given to people suffering from kidney failure and chronic nerve disease. The native peoples of the northern regions of Russia and Afghanistan use a similar rock secretion (mumiyo) from their mountains.

Looking into amazing potential of monoatomic elements I can't help but mention the platinum based minerals that are not really in anyone's diet today. These include rhodium, iridium, indium, ruthenium, osmium, platinum, gold, palladium and silver. Today it's possible to find these as supplements and I advise angstrom size, if available. These minerals, I believe, can help propel us into the next level of consciousness. Each are taken in different amounts, quantities and times. So if you intend on supplementing with these minerals - try something interesting and dissolve these minerals in a powder form into some filtered or spring water and then water your plants you intend to eat with them. This is a wonderful way to obtain these minerals, as the plants will absorb the minerals transferring them to you in a bioavailable format. Try it with wheatgrass!

Back to Fruit

The best way to get minerals is to simply eat fruit. Fruit trees derive their nutrients through the soil and rain finally being distributed into the fruit itself. This is nature's way of mineralizing us and probably the best out of them all. Nothing is more natural nor easier than letting nature take its course. We reap the benefits of growing and consuming produce with consideration of Mother Earth (and Father God).

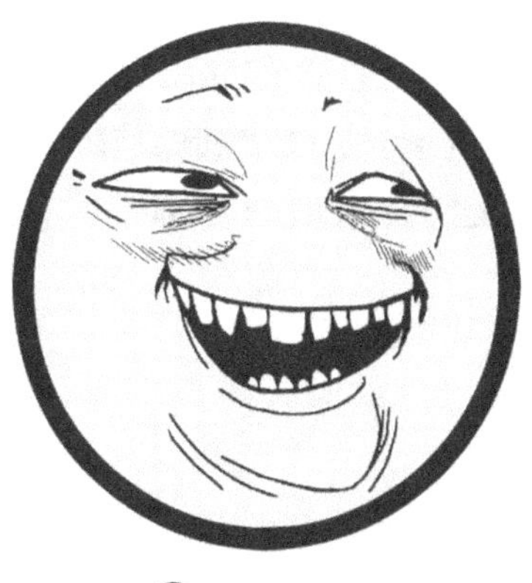

SUGAR

Glycemic Index (GI)

The Glycemic Index is an index of which foods turn into how much sugar in the blood. This is an important factor in anyone wanting to live a long healthy life and everyone should learn what foods spike insulin. Carbohydrates can screw up our metabolic system because it raises our blood glucose levels that makes us produce extra insulin & over time can lead to pre-diabetic state or even full blown Type 2 diabetes.

Under no circumstance are high fructose corn syrup, or agave nectar to be used by diabetics. The processing methods and resulting products are dangerous to the health of everyone, but especially diabetics, as it pertains to blood sugar.

A great tip for anyone who can't beat the sugar habit is to add some fiber to the meal as it slows sugar intake down and keep insulin at bay.

Honey

Honey is my favorite food. And to think, it's just bee hurl! Ha ha ha. But really, what an amazing liquid it is. Honey contains a wider array of nutrients than ANY other food. Some say not enough to sustain a person for very long, but I live on honey for long periods of time without anything else. Throughout history honey has been seen as a holy food.

The Qur'an mentions rivers of honey in paradise.

"And thy Lord taught the bee to build
its cells in hills, on trees
and in men's habitations...
there issues from within their bodies
a drink of varying colors,
wherein is healing for mankind.
Verily in this is a sign
for those who give thought."

Honey is used in memorial celebration by Buddhists in India. It is offered to monks as commemoration for when Buddha made an offering of peace. Buddha retreated into the wilderness and there a monkey brought him honey to eat.

Honey is mentioned in the bible 73 times!!! It is said to have sustained John the Baptist as his major food group along with locust beans (carob pods).

The most amazing thing about honey to me is that it's great before a workout, because the carbohydrates are utilized by the body immediately for energy.

Honey can be taken for reasons such as medical & health benefits like antiseptic, antibacterial, antimicrobial, anti-fungal, bleeding & wound care. And it is by far the best natural preservative for anything in the world. I use it for storage of my herbs. The 2000+ year old honey that was found in the Great Pyramid of Giza is still edible. I find it the best food to take when you want to fast or feel full in a hurry.

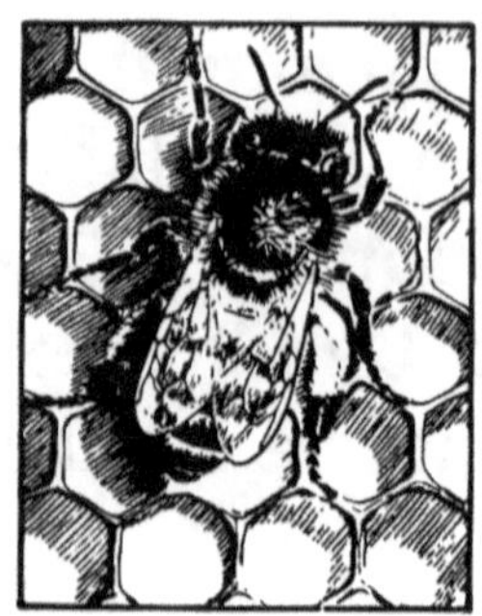

As Good as Gold

Honey, like salt was used to pay taxes in Rome instead of gold. And in Egypt, honey could be traded for ox or donkeys. Take honey away from a bear and you're in a heap of trouble. Bears will literally travel miles if they pick up a sent of honey.

One of the best aspects of honey is that it contains more enzymes than any other food known. Raw wild honey is even low on the Glycemic Index. The Glycemic Index of truly unheated honey is around 40 for some varieties and 55 for the average. It is only when heated that honey becomes extra sugary. The best for diabetics are acacia & tupelo. These are all quite different. Tupelo is gathered from the white tupelo trees that grow along the rivers of the Florida panhandle. Acacia honey is very similar to these but much harder to find and produce. These two kinds of honey have less glucose as opposed to the fructose content of most commercial honeys which are 31% glucose.

Honey can be harvested from soy and corn pollen and I would advise against this GMO pollinated source.

Only two calories of sugar enter into the bloodstream per minute with honey as compared to ten calories with other sugars. One of the sugars in honey (fructose) fuels the brain, which is the most energy demanding organ. The brain can burn up to twenty times the fuel of any other cell in the body. We become exhausted after having to concentrate for a lengthy period. That's why we often hear that mental exhaustion is worse than physical exhaustion. The brain needs glucose to survive, however glucose occupies a large amount of storage space and there is no room for it in the brain. And the liver is the only organ that can both store and release glucose into the circulation. This is why looking after your liver glycogen amount is crucial. Ensuring that the liver and the brain are well provided for both in the day and at night is critical. Any fall in blood glucose is detrimental for the brain.

What I find inspiring to read is that we burn an amazing 70% fat during rest, 35% during low level exercise, 20% during moderate exercise, and a low 10% during intense exercise. During sleep we should burn fats. I find honey to be amazing for fat burning as it stimulates the metabolism. Try taking one tablespoon before bedtime. The liver must deliver 10 grams of glucose every hour: 6.5 to the brain, 3.5 to the kidneys and red blood cells. This glucose encourages your body to burn up fats. But since the liver capacity is only 75 grams - most people go to bed with a depleted liver.

When the liver is not fueled prior to bed, we release stress hormones from the adrenal glands which raise our heart rate and blood pressure. When the adrenal glands are activated and adrenal hormones are overproduced, it can lead to conditions such as heart disease, osteoporosis, obesity, diabetes, poor immune function, depression and other distressing health problems. So instead of burning fat, adrenal hormones degrade muscle and bone.

The author of the "Hibernation Diet" believed that this diet is not only to a healthy weight but unlocking energy resources you never know you had. It essentially aims to encourage people to reap the benefit of their body's own natural recovery system and optimize their recovery biology or fat burning biology, as explicitly outlined above.

Some vegans and pure raw foodists look upon honey as simply bee vomit, and those people are sadly mistaken. Honey not only has the most powerful electrical force found in nature, but it also supplies nutrients necessary for healthy tissue regeneration and stimulates the growth of new blood capillaries. Honey draws lymph out to the cells while absorbing moisture and providing an anti-inflammatory action. It contains Vitamins A, B complex, C, D, E, and K, beta-carotene, minerals, and more enzymes than any other food ever tested in the world.

Honey acts as a natural antibiotic while promoting the growth of beneficial bacteria. Honey promotes the mobility of joint tissue along with the ability to pull calcium into the bones. Honey is a natural antioxidant source. Drinking a mixture of four tablespoons of honey per sixteen ounces of water increases antioxidant levels in the blood.

Honey does not cause cavities like sugar and actually helps fight ulcers. It is a quick source of Energy - fructose and glucose are absorbed directly and easily into the blood. Glucose is what runs our brain and since our brain uses 80% of all calories burned it is vital in the health of this organ and its ability to function properly. Honey provides greater endurance and is one of the most effective forms of carbohydrate to ingest just prior to exercise.

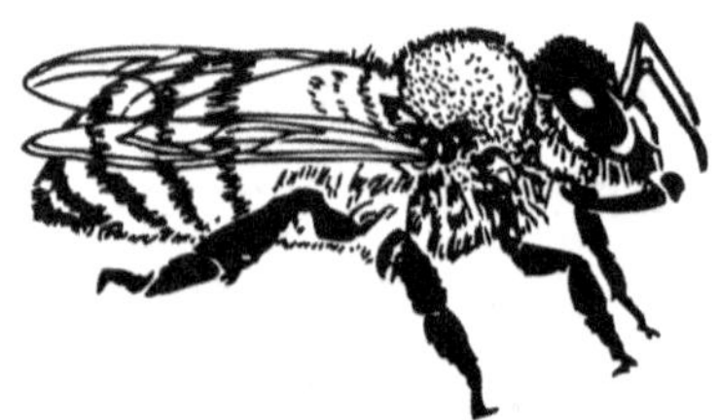

Try to obtain local honey to your area as it can also help you acclimate to your surroundings and help with pollen allergies. Wildflower is often times the best choice because one might not have any idea what pollen they are allergic to. Its best to not mix various kinds of honey together but rather stick to a single kind, the body processes each form of minerals in the honey differently.

As I have discussed, enzymes are the body's life force and fountain of youth. Enzymes are the essential biochemical units regulating and coordinating all life. Only with enzymes is life possible. Enzymes are the missing link to radiant vitality. Enzymes allow life and are the most important nutrient for longevity there is. Vitamins and minerals are only activated by enzymes. Aging is the slow depletion of enzymes from the body. Unheated honey is one of the few foods you can ingest where you are getting a surplus of amylase. This is the enzyme that breaks down sugars and carbohydrates.

More Notes on Honey

A secret most don't know is that most things with a raw label are still heated above 150 degrees. By law they are allowed to do this without repercussion, this is why I advise looking for "unheated" honey rather than raw, as this is truly the best you can obtain. It should not be completely runny or watery. Instead unheated honey will pour slower like a thick syrup or even be completely solid and unable to pour.

I advise honey for everyone except when doing certain cleanses. Because honey is sugar, one can essentially keep feeding fungus if one is out of balance with Candida or other yeast infections. The same tactic used in rat poison can apply to parasite cleansing. If one is doing a parasite cleansing consider using honey as bait with other such herbs as wormwood, quissa, male fern, clove, gentian, false unicorn, graviola, garlic, turmeric etc. The parasites will try to obtain the sugar and as they eat it – they also ingest their own poison.

Honey should be something vegans should adapt to their diet because nothing helps the environment more than supporting local bee farmers. Bees help to produce the very air we breathe by keeping the plants and the trees we need to supply us all with oxygen alive. Looking to a sustainable future, a disservice is done when honey and bee products are overlooked as nutritive. Without supporting bees we will learn the hard way how important these helpers truly are to our future. One cannot ever find a replacement for these mighty workers.

I would not advocate something that I do not fully endorse or do myself, and I fully recommend that one seriously try to obtain the best raw honey obtainable and incorporate it into your diet. Mixing herbs and superfoods into the mix is a fun experience and a great way to pack in high amounts of nutrients into a small amount of food.

Rarely do I go into this much detail about honey, even though I consider it the most perfect food. I personally live on almost 100% honey diet, with the rest being spirulina, herbs, water and some fruit. I would estimate that I only take into a daily caloric count of around 500 on average. And I attribute my powerful calorie restriction ability to the fact that honey is a powerhouse of pure nutrition and ORMUS (more on ORMUS in another book!).

My Last Words on Honey

- "Hundreds of mice have demonstrated that pollen is a complete food and that it is possible to let several successive generations be born and live without the least sign of distress while nourishing them exclusively on pollen."

- "Bee pollen contains all the essential components of life; it corrects the failings due to deficient or unbalanced nutrition."

- "Bee pollen stimulates the production of hemoglobin . . . we have noted counts rising to 4 to 4.5 million. The large proportions of free amino acids, especially methionine, a specific medicine for the liver, explains the favorable action of bee pollen on that organ."

- Honey is the only food that if stored right never goes bad.

- Honey was used for many topical beautification techniques throughout history. Cleopatra of Egypt regularly took honey & milk baths to maintain her youthfulness. Madame du Barry, mistress of King Louis XV, used honey as a facial mask. The Aztecs used honey and clay for a cleansing mask and skin revitalization. Chinese women have a tradition of using a blend of orange seed oil and honey to remedy blemishes and applying honey to wounds is a wonderful healing agent.

- There are over 300 kinds of honey in the US alone!

- Honey has more enzymes than any food ever tested and rare antioxidants like pinocembrine are only found in honey.

- Honey is the only food that can be found worldwide in all cultures and mentioned in every religion as one of the most sacred spiritual foods one can eat.

"Bee pollen contains all the essential elements for healthy tissue and may well prove to be the natural cancer preventive all the world is seeking."

"To my knowledge, there is no better and more complete natural nutrient than honeybee pollen."

Ernesto Contreas, M.D.
cancer specialist

HEALTH ISSUES

*"So I am living without fats,
without meat,
without fish,
but am feeling quite well this way."*

Albert Einstein

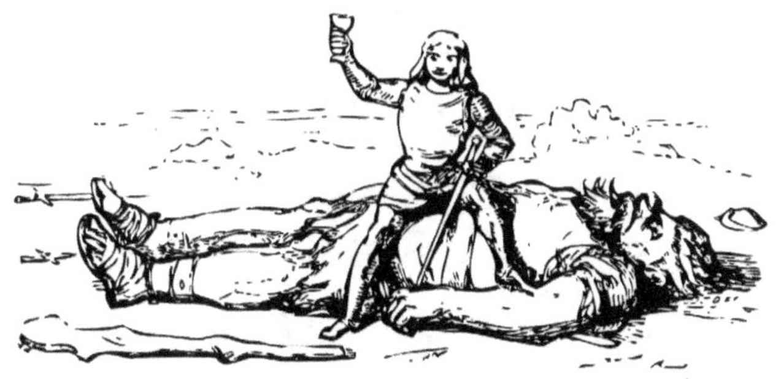

VITALITY

I have more energy and focus than anyone you will ever meet. I have the ability to sit, work, write books like this, and then run to the gym and work out for hours straight. The mind and body work together, neglect one, and the other fails.

I am annoyed of seeing sick and tired people when they have the ability to change it. There's so much worthless propaganda and media selling weight loss pills saying, "Sit on your ass and loose the weight!" I'm here to tell you that's an outright lie. Most programs today have been designed by someone who knows nothing about nutrition. Yet they somehow came up with a get rich quick idea, and through smart mass marketing influence people into thinking it's a good thing. These quacks don't know you or care about you or your health. They want results though; Results that bulk up their wallet!

I hope that I'm wrong about this, but that is what I am seeing in most of the health world.

Energy comes from enthusiasm. No matter what you do in life, the more enthused you are about something, the more of your time and effort you're going to put into it. Become enthused about life and then you will find a renewed energy for doing the things you have been missing out on.

First off, GET MOVING… Set the remote on top of the TV so that every time you want to change the channel you actually have to get up to physically do it. It's amazing how lazy we have become that if the remote isn't within reach we cuss and get angry and try to use "the force" to pull it to us.

I promise you, that the more you start exercising and moving during the day the more energy you are going to have, and topped with a diet consisting of raw living foods that digest easily, your energy levels will be off the charts. Not one day goes by where the energy that flows through my veins doesn't feel like a surge of electricity, powering me through the day.

Old Dogs Can Learn

Some say that the older we become, the harder it is to adapt a new lifestyle. I disagree with this. You CAN teach an old dog new tricks. It's all about willingness and I'm here to tell you that life is far from over even when you wake up and feel weak and sore from the day before. The fatigue and soreness are all just symptoms of a mental and emotional connection to things like diet, sleep and stress. All of these things are mental and YOU have influence over them. I promise you, that by the time you are done reading this chapter, you will have a new outlook on ways to change your life.

My parents have always been in pretty good health, but they have not had the best diet. My mom recently had her cholesterol checked at the doctors and was 279 (LDL cholesterol). They wanted to put her on statin (cholesterol reducing) drugs. I asked the doctor for some time to correct this problem, but they said in three weeks she will be tested again to decide what meds she needs to be on.

For three weeks I had her walking daily around Las Vegas with me and taking just two supplements: polycosanol (23mg) and red yeast rice (600mg). Her diet shifted from eating chicken and dairy to mostly vegetarian. Out of all the animal products I only allowed cheese in her diet. Most people don't realize that all cholesterol comes from animal products. I also let her eat as many avocados as she liked because they raise HDL levels which in turn lower the bad cholesterol LDL.

After three weeks had passed I went back to the doctors with her. Her test results showed cholesterol levels below 180. The doctors were confused about this asked her what she took to make this happen. She told them that I directed her through a diet change and exercise. They told her that diet does not affect the numbers that much and they became very irritated at me.

Needless to say, I cost them money by not having another person on life-long symptom-suppressing drugs. It did not put a smile on their faces. My mom is still tested every four months with checkups and every time has better and better blood, and it's all because of diet. Regardless whether or not someone says, "It doesn't matter what you eat," the numbers don't lie. You ARE what you eat.

And we make a decision about our own heath with every bite we take. Don't dig your own grave spoonful by spoonful. It's slow and painful, and unnecessary.

If you could follow me to the gym, you would see me doing dead lifts and other exercises with ease. I'm not trying to brag. I am making the point that a person on a raw diet for years and years does not lose vitality and energy, but gains it in abundance. As a matter of fact, I'm off to the gym right now. Bye.

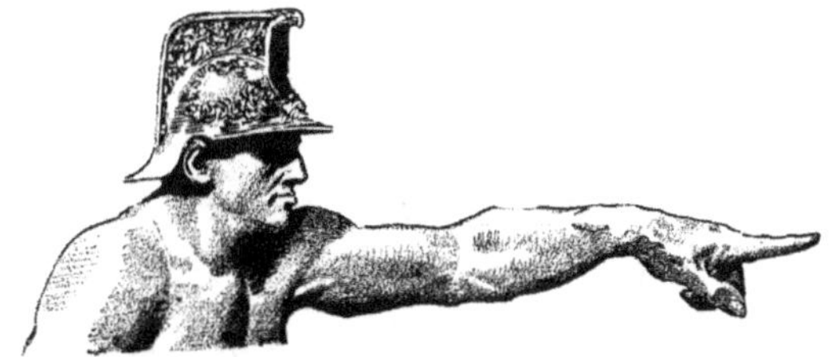

Longevity

Longevity is possible.

Dean Wu Chung-chieh of the department of Education at Minkuo University, China, discovered records in the Imperial Chinese chronicles dated 1777 notes about Li Ching-yung who had been honored for being 100 years old. He went on to relate that the 1877 annals reported the same Li Ching-yung celebrating his second anniversary, living in Kai-shen, Szechwan Province. Li was born May 1677 making him 256 years old when he died in 1933. The article "Tortoise-Pigeon-Dog", from the May 15, 1933 issue of Time reports his history and his secrets to longevity. He supposedly lived on mostly fruit and plants and herbs.

It is recorded in the parish register of St. Leonard's, Shoreditch that Thomas Carn died in 1588 in the reign of Queen Elizabeth at age 207. He was born in 1381, in the reign of Richard II and lived in the reigns of ten sovereigns.

Thomas Parr was an English man who was often referred to Old Tom Parr supposedly lived for 152 years. He supposedly was born in 1483 and joined the army around 1500. He married when he was 80 years old and had two children, a son and a daughter, both of whom died in infancy. Allegedly he had an affair and a child born out of wedlock around 100 years old. After the death of his first wife, he married again at the alleged age of 122. He attributed his long life to his vegetarian diet: green cheese, onions, coarse bread, buttermilk or mild ale (cider) on special occasions, and no smoking.

His recipe for long life was reputed to be:

*"Keep your head cool by temperance
and your feet warm by exercise.
Rise early,
go soon to bed,
and if you want to grow fat [prosperous]
keep your eyes open
and your mouth shut."*

When news of his age spread, 'Old Parr' became a national celebrity. He was painted by Rubens and Van Dyke. In 1635, he was brought him to London to meet Charles I. The king asked Parr what he had done that was greater than any other man, and Parr replied that he had performed penance (for his affair) at the age of 100. While in London, he was treated as a spectacle. But it was supposedly the change in food and environment apparently caused his death. He is buried in Westminster Abbey.

Katherine Fitzgerald who was referred to as "the old Countess of Desmond Katherine Fitzgerald," lived to the age of 140 years. Lady Desmond was reported to have been capable, just before her death, of walking four to five miles every week to her local market, and it was said that all her teeth had been renewed a few years earlier. The story is she died after falling from a tree where she picked cherries for breakfast. What a way to go.

Marie-Louise Fébronie Chassé Meilleur died of a blood clot at age 117 in April 1998 in Corbeil, Ontario, and her oldest living daughter, Gabrielle Vaughan, was 90 years old. She was said to be a vegetarian. Even as of 2008, the current longevity record holder Jeanne Calment died at the age of 122. We still see cases of longevity right in front of us.

Norman W. Walker

Dr. Norman W. Walker born January 28, 1867 is recognized throughout the world as one of the most authoritative students of life, health and nutrition. For almost 70 years, Dr. Walker researched man's ability to live a longer, healthier life. He was his own example of achieving vibrant health through proper thought, diet and body care. The books written by Dr. Walker have been printed every year since the mid-1930s. Over the decades these books have been in print, other researchers have confirmed Dr.

Walker's findings. Never have any of his findings been proven wrong. Well past his 100th birthday, Dr. Walker was growing his own produce in the blistering heat of Arizona and still doing research on food chemistry and its effect on the human body. He passed on June 6, 1985 at the young age of 118.

Eat Less

Caloric restriction is the only true modern day scientific approach where the study on humans & animals alike shows potential for achieving longevity and is what I personally practice. I believe caloric restriction with low Glycemic Index (GI) diet that balances your intestinal flora, keeps the system strong and disease at bay. If you do consume higher amounts of calories then you must burn them off via exercise. If caloric intake is not burned, it is stored and converted to fat and that promotes death.

We are highly adaptable creatures. We are an open system. By this I mean that one could eat junk food for twenty years and then with a simple shift in diet and consciousness, one can turn around all aspects of their internal system. The body can naturally regenerate itself, if given time and proper nutrients. It is not what one has not done that causes deficiencies. It was has done in excess that has the most detrimental effect.

Cutting down on your protein is most important because our bodies cannot store access amino acids. If they are not utilized by muscle they enter our blood stream and make our system highly acidic, causing special harm to our liver and kidneys.

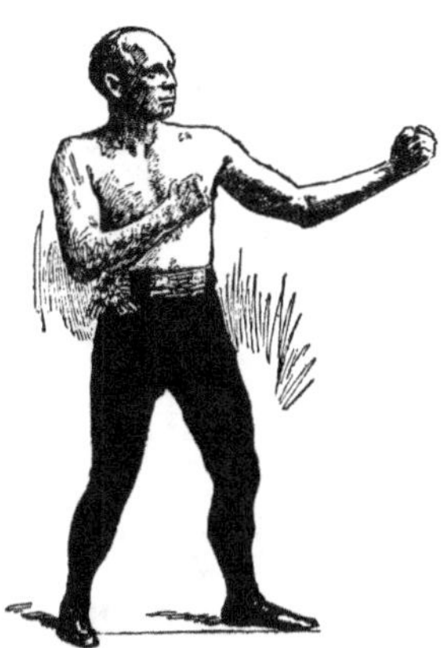

PHYSIQUE AND MUSCLE

I have luckily always been naturally very thin. Working out for me is not a hindrance because I have made it a part of my lifestyle. It's like breathing; it's just something I have to do. I never consume breakfast, I feel best on consumption of carbohydrates through fruit. I lean towards papaya and seeded grapes for hydration and figs and dates for meals with hemp, walnut, almonds or Brazil nuts (all soaked & sprouted). When I am unable to find any of the above items organic, then I just live on honey till the season rolls around that I can obtain organic produce again.

I live in the desert, so finding wild foods can be near impossible. But there are a lot of wild date palms, carob & olive trees, aloe vera &

herbs if you know where to look. So even in the desert – you can live a raw life. Imagine how much more live food you can find if you live in the mountains, plains or by the sea!

Building Muscle

The top muscle building vegetables are kale, sprouts and cabbage. Kale has rich mineral content and very high in antioxidants & minerals because their soil is usually richer than normal greens. I like to blend celery, cabbage with a few leaves of kale and lemon. Blended or juiced vegetables and greens are better than the whole form, because most of us don't take the time to chew our food properly. On top of that, it is hard to break down plant cellulose in the mouth and digestive tract. Blending or juicing helps that process to extract nutrition.

The top seed for muscle growth is undoubtedly hemp seeds. It is the most usable protein in the plant kingdom. They contain no enzyme inhibitors thus require no sprouting or preparation. The total protein content of hemp seed is about 65% of the globular protein edestin, which closely resembles the globulin found in human blood plasma. Containing the all known 21 amino acids, Hemp seeds are an absolute must for anyone trying to gain the most size on a raw vegan diet.

The best fruit for muscle growth are figs & dates. Dates are a bit high in sugar but some varieties are higher in fiber than others, thus the GI is much lower. I tend to lean towards all foods lower glycemic. The fig is higher in fiber and also well suited for strength. Some primates live on a diet consisting 80% of figs. These foods tend to be higher in calories than other fruits, but supply great nutrient benefits to a system undergoing physical stress. I always say eat what grows near you, so if you live in a desert search for dates, if you are near the coast look for figs.

The food closest to whey protein is bee pollen. Pollen, like whey, is broken down into free form amino acids that the body doesn't have to do any conversion with. This makes pollen the most easily digestible protein around, and unlike whey it's not acidic forming in the body and is biodegradable. Make sure to take bee pollen with honey as they work synergistically.

Training in the Raw

I never wanted a huge body builder's physique, because it's not natural. But I do like to carry muscle around, because it's a nice motivating factor to encourage people to change their diet. If I look too skinny and scrawny it might just scare people off of the raw life. 63% of America is obese. Because of this, the average skinny person looks like they have an eating disorder as opposed to just plain healthy. We live in a society where looks are a major factor. You know this is true just looking at any magazine cover at a local grocery store. So to be a good example of a raw food diet, it seems logical to look physically fit standing next to an average person.

Because I naturally have a fast metabolism and also eat raw, it is hard to keep muscle on. So I keep fit weight lifting five or six days a week. I find that on a raw vegan diet muscle recovery is equal to or greater than on a typical diet. This makes one able to work out more often and with heavier weights. This is not always a good thing, because the body grows while in a state of rest. Since the body does not feel sore, one tends to over train and not grow as much muscle as one would like. This is where smart training becomes much more important than standard training methods.

I personally find that spending less time in the gym but training with focus and intent is much more important than how long you were at the gym. It's not about telling people "yeah I spend six hours a day working out." It's about what you do with the time in the gym, and more does not necessarily mean better. Muscle doesn't take much effort to tear, and tearing your muscles down is what creates the micro tears that create growth. This is why recovery is important and why it doesn't truly matter how long you spend in the gym.

I use short and sweet workouts, oftentimes only spending a little more than an hour in the gym with 15 minutes of that stretching. Remember that the muscles in the body break down relatively fast, especially using heavy weights. The secret to growth isn't about using as much weight as you can possibly push, rather it's all about tearing muscle down.

Weight Training

The body has no idea what weight it's pushing, meaning it doesn't know the difference between ten or one hundred pounds it only knows stress or resistance. So to push one hundred pounds one time with sloppy form and almost passing out is more harmful than beneficial. Rather one should use proper form, with less weight which builds the body much more efficiently than how much weight you do use.

I suggest that you always keep transitioning your weights, as the body is an amazing thing. It adapts to almost anything, and even the stress of weights the body becomes used to. This is why personal trainers keep their jobs, because they know that after a short time, people stop getting results on their own, because they never change their workouts. Often times after a month of similar exercises, I change my routine completely. This never lets the body adapt and keeps it growing. So if body building or just muscle gain is your goal, you must constantly change your routine to find benefit.

Remember, while exercise and rest restore muscles, proper nutrition also plays a key role. The most important foods and supplements that I recommend you get on immediately are: bee pollen, figs, grapes, hemp seeds, Brazil nuts and honey. As far as supplements are concerned, internal and transdermal magnesium chloride and internal magnesium citrate are the best for muscle recovery. Now we all know about protein. And America is obviously the highest consumer of this diet, which is a concern. For higher consumption of protein, digestive enzymes such as protease and papain become another important supplement for your fitness goals. I do not recommend any of the commercially available fat burners, whey proteins, meal replacements, or other 'ingestible' fitness products. Often they are filled with all sorts of dangerous unhealthy ingredients such as fillers, binders, preservatives, and indigestible gluten proteins.

Brain Health

The brain is the most amazing organ of the body. Out of all the millions of nerves in the body, the brain doesn't have a single one. The brain is essentially made of fat, and the body protects it the best it can from debris & foreign proteins by only allowing one platelet of blood pass through the blood brain barrier out of 240 platelets.

Besides the brain controlling everything from emotions, perception and learning, to physical skills and sensory systems, from blood regulation to fluid balance, the brain does more than science will ever understand. The brain only works at less than fraction of its total functional capability. Interpret this as you will and imagine what our true capacity to achieve can be. So many preternatural phenomena may be possible: telekinesis, multi-dimensional sight, precognition, etc.

The brain once hindered is the hardest organ to fix because it's the hardest to gets nutrients to and from. The brain being fat can store toxins the same way body fat tissue can, this is why most people get headaches over and over and nothing seems to alleviate them.

The best thing about adopting a raw vegan diet is that from that point on the brain is only being fed the right nutrients; nutrients that don't contain harmful viruses, tumors, bacterial, fungal or parasitic organisms that can corrode, deteriorate or eat the brain. Of course parasites can still be on produce, so you have to wash with hydrogen peroxide or Apple Cider vinegar (ACV). But since you will not be cooking, the risk for harmful elements in your food and the amount of heavy metals in your diet will dramatically decrease which is a huge step in longevity. Most major ailments that degenerate the brain come from heavy metal toxicity and chemicals from our environment.

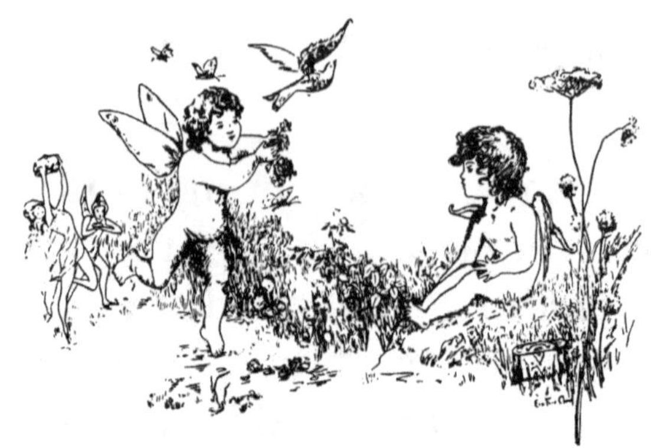

AUTISM

The study of autism is relevant to everyone. A child with autism is considered to have a brain development disorder that inhibits social communication or interactions. Autism has tripled since the 1980s and is known for causing anti-social behavior and inability to function properly later in life. Autism affects males over females at a ratio of 4:1, predominantly because of testosterone. Autism is different from most diseases, as it is affected by hormones and brain stimulation.

The reason Autism is so hard to catch is because the symptoms of it all occur before a child is three years old. Some believe that it's vaccine related, but no scientific evidence is shown to prove this. But we'll see more about that in a bit…

Autistic behavior includes repetitive behavior like head rocking and waving arms in air & rocking back and forth, as well as bad focus, short attention span, bodily harm, and arrangement of items certain ways. Contrary to common belief, autistic children do not prefer to be alone. Autistic infants show delayed onset of babbling and as they age they make less frequent & diverse babbling.

Children tend to respond less to their own name the older they get, and display moderately less attachment security than usual.

Treatment for this is not as simple or correctable with diet as other issues. Autism usually occurs from missing the crawling stage of life, where a child never learns the cross lateral pattern. Motor development is crucial to a child, and unlike dyslexia the brain of a child with autism has a brain structure that is not protected by the blood brain barrier. Wheat legumes, beans and dairy (other than mother's milk) can be detrimental as this blood brain barrier is not yet functional or protective to the developing brain.

When large indigestible proteins like casein, gliadin and glutenin from foods get into the brain, they affect the vagus nerve (ability to read emotions) and cerebellum (motor skills). In the last few decades the autism rate in America has gone from 1 in 2500 children to 1 in 150! Why?

One amazing study was showing the heavy link of mercury & led in the brains of all children with autism. In a report released in mid-July, the Environmental Working Group (EWG) identified a total of 287 industrial chemicals, pollutants, and other contaminants in the blood of the umbilical cords of ten newborn babies. Of those compounds, EWG stated that 180 cause cancer in humans or animals, 217 are toxic to the brain and nervous system of humans or animals, and 208 can cause birth defects in humans and animals. Included among the chemicals were seven high-toxicity pesticides, some of which have been illegal to use or produce in the United States for over thirty years.

Some of the chemicals found in umbilical cord blood include mercury, a potent neurotoxin; polyromantic hydrocarbons, which have been linked to cancer; organochlorine pesticides like DDT, hexachlorobenzene, dieldrin, and aldrin, all of which are known to cause cancer, interfere with reproductive development, or both; and PBDE flame retardants, commonly found in household dust and thought to adversely affect brain development and the thyroid.

Vaccines and Mercury

One third of most vaccines contain mercury and most kids today that have autism are because kids systems can't throw off this metal and because it causes inflammation of the brain. The heavy metals are stored in the brain fat. There is not one case of autism present in the Amish community because they do not allow vaccines.

It is strange to me that mercury is against the law to handle or take to school, but yet they add it to your teeth in fillings. And the toxins dymarysol or amarisol in mercury are not ever taken out even by distillation. They also tell you that the virus in the vaccine is dead but this is not true, they show up later on in life attached to the spinal column completely alive. Also, every case of an autistic child has live measles in their brains or in their spinal fluid.

A good example of how truly hard vaccines are on the system can be found in a book written when vaccines were introduced into the aborigine tribes of Africa called Every Other One. It is an accounting of a true event where aborigine tribes were vaccinated and every other one died.

Correcting Autism

The number one action one must take in correcting this condition is to kill the viruses that perpetuate it through unbalanced intestinal flora.

Organic virgin coconut oil has the ability to destroy lipid (fat based) viruses, which is ideal for detoxifying the brain and spinal column. I recommend feeding three to seven tablespoons of coconut oil per day. Cook exclusively with coconut oil, foregoing all other oils except for extra virgin olive oil in moderation. Have the child eat the coconut straight from the spoon or add it to smoothies, juices, cereals, desserts, and other food or drink.

In the first five years of a child's life much can be restored if caught early enough. Most research today shows that after a child has reached a certain age they are unable to recover because of brain damage. A humic formula of fulvic acids (X1) has been shown to pull out mercury with good results.

EDTA is weak but also shows promise for mercury detoxification.

Sun chlorella with cilantro can also help to chelate mercury and eliminate it through the urine. These foods, when chewed in a salad or other savory food help to pass the blood brain barrier and help to bind heavy metals.

NCD liquid Zeolites are an excellent heavy metal chelation method.

Try supplementation with niacin (B3) which helps circulation and stimulates extra blood to the brain along with a powerful fat called lecithin. B3 is bioavailable in rice bran solubles (one to three tablespoons per day), bee pollen (one to three teaspoons per day), and royal jelly (one quarter to one teaspoon per day).

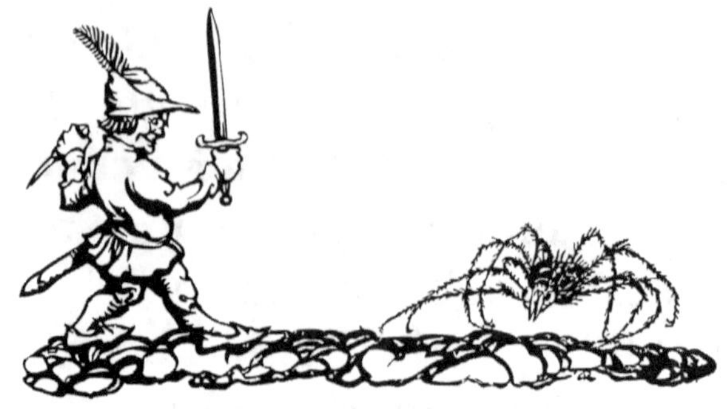

PARASITES!

I can't think of a more important chapter than this one. Parasites truly are the enemy within. Jesus referred to parasites as Satan!

There are over 300 varieties of parasites in America alone that can be ingested through the air we breathe, water we drink, food we eat and even from simply walking barefoot or petting an animal. Most of us have them and would never know, as doctors themselves have no idea how to even test for most of the different varieties. There are a few ways to kill all the different types, below are the specific outlines for specific breeds. I am a huge fan of herbs and I myself use them for a parasite cleanse, this takes a while longer but is also more effective in the long run and better for your body.

Fish and meats all have parasites today, to high consumption of these foods really makes the body more susceptible to these foreign invaders. Eating fish will eventually lead to a thiaminase deficiency & most likely heavy metal poisoning & parasites. This is a fact. Meat unless cooked is very blood filled, fat filled piece of protein harboring many bad bacteria & parasites. It is very hard for the body to process, since all assimilation of nutrients are absorbed in the small intestine. Someone eating meat is digesting nothing but rotten flesh. Since it takes many hours for such high amounts of protein to reach this area of the body, its best to just not consume such a burdensome food that

1) lacks enzymes,

2) contains bacteria, parasites

3) forms HeteroCyclic Amines (HCA carncinogens) when cooked,

4) has no fiber, and plus,

5) way over 60% of cows today have leukemia!

Yuk. It's never smart to eat meat.

<u>Symptoms of Infection</u>

Parasites have a list of symptoms, but remember that you are their host. They don't want to harm you, or even let you know they are there most of the time. They are living off of what you feed them, so their intent is to stay hidden and breed and because we are symbiotic organism ourselves, our body is at war with them and we have no idea. By the time most people realize they have them, it is sometimes too late, as they can breed very fast. Consider the case with house pets. The main cause of death to both dog and cats is a parasite known as heart worm.

When symptoms do arise, they are usually diarrhea, anemia, headaches, fatigue, mood swings, bowel problems, weight management issues, insomnia, or intestinal pains. The list is actually much larger, and parasites are often the main culprits behind those listed. The most astounding thing about most major disease, deaths and even all forms are cancer are that they are all related to parasites!

Parasites poison us through their metabolic waste and it is probably one of the main reasons for lack of sleep because their urine is pure ammonia. Amoebae also release an enzyme that causes ulcers. Similar to fungus, parasites burrow into organs and make a mess of things. They steal minerals & amino acids as food to live. They can erode damage or block certain organs by lumping together in balls or tumors. They can be mistaken for cancer tumors, and travel into the brain, heart and lungs. Endo Limax Nana is a parasite that has been found to eat the calcium off our bones causing forms of arthritis. Entamoeba Histolytica can get into the liver, the lungs and the brain.

Today scientists are even relating seizures with a parasite that could be burrowing it way into the brain. Amazing that pets can even pass on worms to their owners. A recent study showed that heart disease and heart attacks may be higher in dog owners, as these owners have had their hearts infected by the worms their pet possessed. This condition has been confirmed by autopsy.

Releasing Parasites

There are several types of intestinal worms. The most common of these are giardia roundworms, toxoplasmosis, pin worms, whipworm thread worms, roundworms, hookworms, flukes & tapeworms. Below I will give cheap simple solutions for each, and the herbs that are best to destroy them.

When you do a parasite cleanse it is important to do it correctly or you will just end up feeding them. A diet high in fruit and sprouted seeds is best. Most people think that the parasites would feast on these foods, but they actually help as flushing agents as they are digested readily fast in comparison to most all other foods.

I suggest starting a colon cleanse program because it's a breeding ground for bacteria & parasites. Parasites breed mostly there and find the warm damp moist area of that region quite pleasing. Before I get into what foods and herbs upset parasites the most, this is probably the fastest creepiest and easiest way to rid them of the colon area. Take castor oil capsules and freeze them. When thoroughly frozen take around 3-6 caps every 24 hours, as these caps in a frozen state don't get absorbed by the stomach but pass right through. By the time they reach the last part of the small intestine they dissolve in the ileum, the last three fifths of the small intestine. Here the digestive tract converts this oil into recinoleic acid, which is harmless to humans but deadly to parasites.

NEVER GIVE CHILDREN 5 years or younger castor oil.

Out of all the whole foods that help expel most kinds of intestinal worms the top of the ladder is coconut. Taking a tablespoon of freshly ground coconut meat throughout the day is amazing. If one does this along with the frozen castor oil capsules, intestinal parasites are sure to be running for their lives in no time.

Colloidal Silver

Colloidal silver is powerful; it kills not only viruses and bacteria, but Parasites alike. Basically, silver just helps the body to clear these pathogens by disabling a specific enzyme that microorganisms need to breathe. When the enzyme is disabled, the microorganism quickly suffocates and dies.

Garlic

Garlic is a cleansing herb that has been used since ancient times. This plant is destructive to parasites. The ancients used to put a clove of garlic in their sandals and as they walked it would become crushed. Thus their skin would absorb the oil and the penetrating oil would enter the blood and carry it to the intestines killing them along its path. But this is mainly for those who cannot consume garlic either because of taste or a late night date!

Because garlic is very harsh internally, I only recommend it 3 days a week at most because of the fact that it is so devastating to bacteria including "good" flora. Perhaps Monday, Wednesday and Friday consume the garlic cloves and relax the rest of the week to allow your good flora to remain strong and vital. On the days in-between consider aloe vera. It is related to the garlic family and contains high amounts of sulfur and polysaccharides.

Carrot

Carrot is useful in the elimination of thread worms in kids as it is offensive to most parasites. A small cup of grated carrot taken every morning, with no other food added to the meal can clear worms quickly. Make sure not to juice carrots, but keep them whole. Once parasites are destroyed, only consume carrots in their whole form or blended, if at all, as they are high in sugar.

Papaya

Round worms are best killed with unripe papayas as they contain an enzyme called papain. Even the seeds are wonderful as they contain a substance called caricin. Add them to a salad for an enjoyable, peppery, spicy taste.

Turmeric

Turmeric kills various parasites as well, like lice and scabies (microscopic parasitic mites that infect the skin). Make a paste and apply it to all the affected areas each day for a couple of weeks or until the problem is gone. For lice, it's also a good idea to boil your clothes and bedding to prevent re-infection. Take turmeric to get rid of other parasites too, especially nematodes. Turmeric contains four anti-parasitic chemicals, each of which is not effective alone, but when combined, they make a strong worm-killing cocktail. This phenomenon is called synergy and you will never find it in any pharmaceutical drugs since they are all isolated chemicals. Only Nature's whole herbs have this advantage.

Nut Milks and Beyond

I use nut milks for extreme conditions of the blood, as pumpkin seeds are great for worms, especially tape. Sprouting the seeds for eight to twelve hours in water, then blending them with three parts water to one part seeds with a small bit of stevia leaf (a green powder – I do not recommend the processed white stevia) or raw honey really does the trick.

Out of all the herbs, foods, cleanses and powders, fasting is actually THE best way to kill parasites. As fasting essentially starves them to death similar to colloidal silver. And I have heard that you can sometimes even force them out by sitting with your behind in a vat of warm milk and honey but I imagine this would be quite scary to visibly see them come out that way!

Diatoms are used as a pool cleaner for fighting algae and parasites and are now made food grade. This essentially cuts the parasite when ingested because they do not have an out shell protecting them. I have yet to feel physical results from taking this supplement, but often times you never do.

Parasite Prevention

Parasites have been found in water-grown vegetables, so they should be washed with 6% vinegar or potassium permanganate for five to ten minutes which kills the encysted metacercariae. This approach is more successful than attempts to halt the consumption of raw vegetables. Buy organic and avoid growing areas with sewage contamination. Consider cooking or steaming water-grown vegetables thoroughly before eating.

Toxoplasmosis is considered to be the third leading cause of death, attributed to food borne illness in the US. Over sixty million adults will carry this parasite, but very few ever have symptoms. This is because like most parasites, our immune system can keep them from causing illness. This parasite is spread most often by a housecat, but again can be traced back to unwashed produce.

Myrrh is a general purpose anti-microbial. This means that it helps the body destroy or resist bacteria, fungi, and viruses. These properties mean that myrrh is classified as a natural anti-bacterial, anti-biotic, anti-fungal, and disinfectant. As a fungicide, Myrrh not only destroys fungi, but it also prevents and combats fungal infection. Myrrh has been shown to eradicated the parasitic flatworm know as fascioliasis and the fluke.

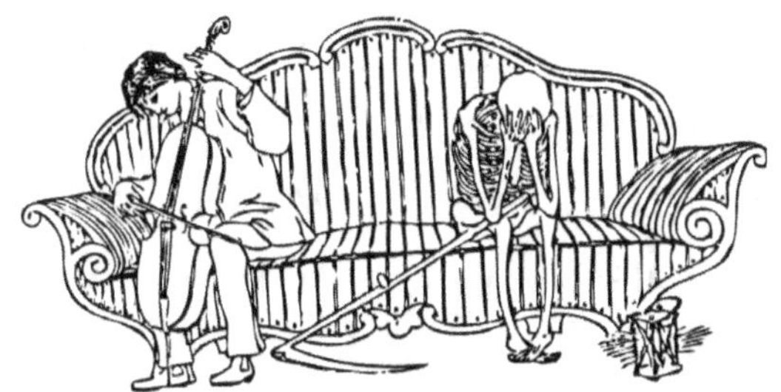

FUNGUS

Fungus and parasites go hand in hand. Once fungus has killed the majority of the intestinal flora it is impossible for the terrain of our gut to ever gain control again without extreme intervention. Fungus problems from vaccines are the worst. Even though the majority of our foods today feed fungus, it is not a problem for people unless they have had vaccinations or are on birth control. I myself trained in martial arts for many years, physically assaulting people with warts, ring worm, skin disease and probably STD's & grappling on mats with athletes foot and worse. Even dandruff is caused by fungus, a tiny fungus called malassezia.

At the peak of my training and professional fighting career, my knees, elbows, wrists and hands were covered in warts, because they were always exposed to the fungus-ridden mats so often. I also had dandruff so I kept my hair short, and athletes foot and nail fungus where my toe nails ended up falling off due to injury. I never wanted put anything on my skin topically, I only want to heal from the inside out. The skin is like a mirror showing me a reflection of what is going on inside my body. But at the peak of my training after being 100% raw for many years now, I have internally fixed all of these problems through diet with the exception of few remaining warts and some minor nail fungus.

Fungus is a diet related disease & often times starts because of our first vaccine. When the immune system is working properly it can simply destroy fungus in its early stages of growth. But when a body on a poor diet comes in contact with fungus, it simply is too weak to fend off the new invader. Now I can train with all my old friends who continue to have all those fungus related ailments that I used to have and never have any new problems arise.

Eating smart by consuming organic living foods helps to flush out and cleanse all debris from the body, creating an alkaline healthy balanced system. Fungus and bacteria thrive in an acid environment and build their own protein layer around themselves to protect themselves from the immune system and then turn into mold. This is incredibly similar to cancer. Cancer cells are surrounded by a thick layer of protein protecting them from your own immune system.

Some foods that we think are healthy actually contribute to fungus growth. Fungus and bacteria love love love sugar. Apples for instance are a breeding ground for a few types of fungus called p.patuluns and a.clavatus and they produce a mycotoxin that can cause allergies called patulin. Oranges and strawberries follow close behind. Most grains contain a fungus because of the way they are stored and even ancient grains like spelt (the great uncle of wheat) contains Ochratoxin A (OTA) is a hazard to man and animals. It is the cause of porcine nephropathy and it is considered carcinogenic.

Peanuts contain over 45 strains of fungi, aflatoxin being the worst and are now illegal to sell in most schools. Corn and similar grains all contain over 25 strains of fungi, usually resulting in a skin rash. Meat, poultry & dairy have the worst reputations. Emmer is the oldest of grains, and even that probably is not resistant to all the new forms of fungus in our Modern environment.

Fungus, bacteria and yeast can survive the strong acid of our stomach and the intestinal track. They work their way through the body, blood, lymph & skin leaving behind them mycotoxin (waste excretion). They consume organic matter, wherever humidity and temperature are sufficient.

Disease is an imbalance of the blood, and fungus plays a major factor in the decline of our health. With proper nutrition and simply using our heads, we stay ahead of the game with an awareness of what's happening around us, to us and inside of us. There are anywhere from four to six pounds of bacteria in the intestinal flora, and even taking antibiotics ONE TIME can send our blood into dysbiosys.

Intestinal dysbiosys is the root cause of disease. 85% of our intestinal flora should be made of good bacteria and 15% is fungal in nature (Candida). This is how it should be in a healthy person, but as our diets are so bad and we have included vaccines to our population we can now have only 15% good bacteria and 85% fungus. This dysbiosys allows fungus to excrete a liquid poison in the blood to kill its enemies and fungus' enemy is our friendly bacteria.

After it has unbalanced our gut flora, fungus moves from the colon where it feeds and eventually moves to the small intestine where it's never supposed to be. Since digestion and assimilation of all the nutrients of our food takes place in the small intestine you can imagine the havoc it can wreck on a system. Now that the fungus is there, it turns sugar into alcohol. Similar to how we make beer, we add sugar to grains. The byproduct is carbon dioxide bubbles. This is why some people when they eat certain carbohydrates like legumes and grains begin to bloat up and get gas, belching and farting.

When the fungus is in the small intestine it begins to drill holes everywhere in the body which show up as rashes, blurry vision, white tongue called thrush, adult acne, rosea, an itchy face, ears etc. One of the first things that happens when fungus overrides the system is you become hypoglycemic, which is a precursor to becoming diabetic! This is all because the fungus disrupts digestion & inhibits mineral absorption. Now that sugar and insulin are not regulated properly guess what the body of a diabetic craves? Sugar, the fuel for the fire itself!

We can actually point the finger at fungus and blame them for such cravings for sugar because we essentially are feeding them by eating these foods. Similar to parasites, they actually make the body crave for certain kinds of foods that are far from the best for us. This is where a diet following a low GI regimen is very important as these foods are low is sugar.

The Critical Link

What is the number one food for fungus? Sugar. What is the major population problem in today's times? Obesity. See the link? Diabetes is an epidemic, and it's exploded since World War II. Most of us never associate disease with a vaccine, because it could take 20 or 30 years before it even shows itself. Fungus like all disease, incubates. And slowly from bottom to top we will wind up with fungus. Before we realize it we are riddled with an almost unstoppable disease that takes an entire lifestyle change to compensate for years of abuse. Unfortunately, many cannot make the transition.

To give you an idea how critical it is to rid the body of fungus, take this into consideration. Most toxins, chemical solvents, environmental hazards, pollution, greenhouse gasses and the like are nothing in comparison to the havoc that mycotoxin excrete in our own bodies. Apples, bananas, corn can contain up to 25 strains of fungi or more specifically aflatoxin (toxic metabolites produced by a variety of molds). Cashews, peanuts, kidney beans & other legumes contain over 40! Grains like barley, rye, wheat etc., and especially dairy, poultry, all meats all contain fungi. Even improperly stored coffee all contain ochratoxin a, which can survive our intestinal track and secrete mycotoxin, which is linked to cancer, kidney disease, and other disorders.

Your personal choice on how much flesh foods are consumed will influence the amount of health obtained.

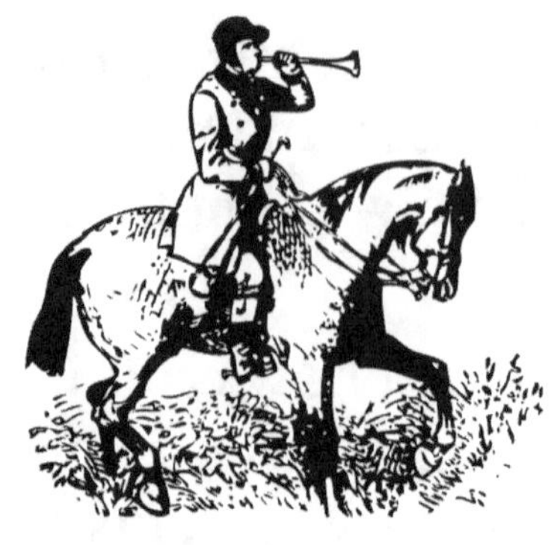

INTESTINAL FORTITUDE

Bowel Disease

Bowel disorders are **absolutely** and **directly** linked right to what you eat. Change your diet and odds are that your bowel problems will get much better and probably disappear. Your health depends on how much of your diet consists of fresh fruit and raw greens and how much fat or protein, especially animal fat or protein. It's that simple.

Indigestible protein consumption in non-raw living foods creates inflammatory bowel disease (IBD). IBD occurs as the lining of the intestinal tract is inflamed. A previously healthy person full of energy can experience nutritional deficiencies followed up by signs and symptoms of bile occlusion and insufficiency. These insufficiencies include a lack of fat-soluble vitamins A, D, E and K. Bile is necessary for fat-soluble vitamin digestion and assimilation.

Symptoms of indigestible proteins, run-away sugars, rancid fat and indications of bile insufficiency from a non-living foods diet include: chronic fatigue syndrome, celiac disease, loss of memory, poor concentration, sore throat, extreme exhaustion, sleep disturbance, headache, pain, swelling, neoplastic conditions, enlarged lymph nodes in the neck and arm pits, abdominal pain, dry mouth, bloating, white leuccoreah discharge, neuritis, weight management challenge, sensory disturbances, cardiovascular disease, immune dysfunction, cystic fibrosis, diabetes, digestive disturbances, mental afflictions, fertility challenges, skin disease, depression, and infections that include increased mucous and secretion of body fluids in the lungs and air-passage ways. Growths in body cavities such as the nasal passages, anus, urethra, as well as hepatitis, cirrhosis of the liver and pancreatitis are all due to an obstruction of bile flow, bile insufficiency and consumption of indigestible proteins.

I believe over 85% of all systemic disease is related to our intestinal track if not more. What's amazing is that some disease can arise from within, without cause of diet but simply from stress-related body tissue.

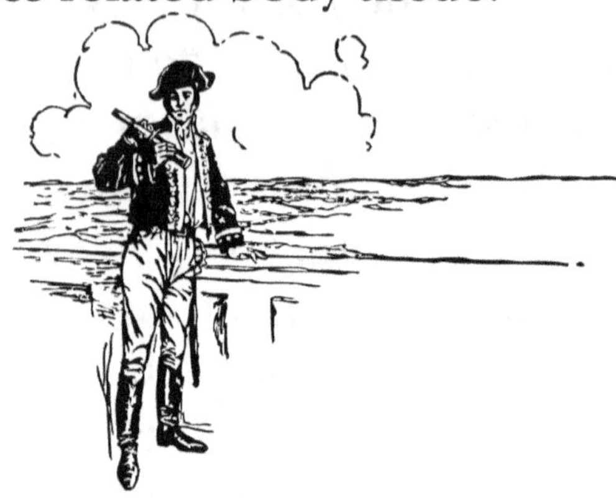

Oxidation and fermentation are all underlying factors to good or bad health. For one to obtain such prevalent health one must flood the body with optimal nutrition and recurring fasting. One cannot have disease and continue with their current routine and expect any different result. We must look at ourselves with a different angle to win the battle of disease in our lives.

Fungus, mold, yeast, bacteria, viruses, parasites & free radical damage (oxidation) all cause aging of the body. Simply eating healthy will not cease this assault breakdown of our system. We need to get involved in this waging war going on inside our bodies whether we like to think of it that way or not. This war is ongoing and it is it all started most likely years ago, as all disease incubates before it shows its ugly head. We have perhaps seen small symptoms, but overlooked them or simply taken something to suppress them. This made the battle inside you into a war and this is much harder to fight. Take steps of action into defeating each of these problems and you will rid the body of all plagues.

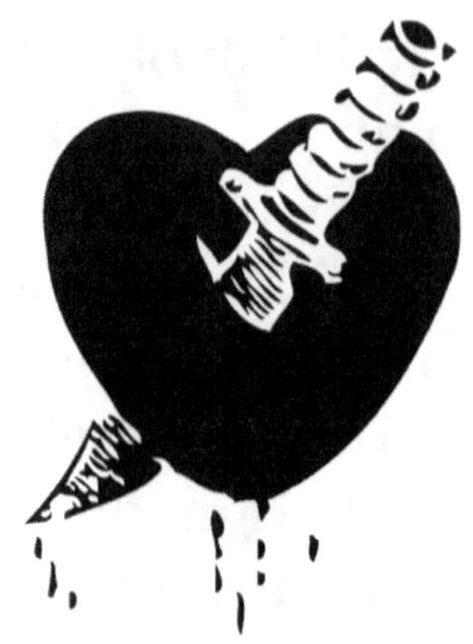

Blood Health

Let's talk dis-ease. 90% of the blood cells inside of our bodies are red blood cells; this majority contributes a great deal to our vitality. Since a red blood cell has an average life of 128 days it's vitally important to keep the diet clean. This directly relates to how long, healthy and strong these blood cells will be. Strong red blood cells keep liver and intestine cells vibrant and able to produce albumin (super transporters). A disease condition can only arise when too much or not enough red blood formation occurs. This can occur from gluttony, poor digestion, or the fungus byproduct nu-toxin.

The quantity of bacteria in our blood and intestines far outnumber the blood cells in our bodies (there are over four to six pounds of bacteria in our gut alone). The maintenance of our health is based on how well our intestinal flora thrive. Our bacteria inside of us can produce everything the body actually requires to live, other than nutrients made within the cell.

Think of a chicken, when it's born as an egg it shows a small amount of nutrients, yet three weeks of incubation there are some 300 times more nutrients. Where did these vitamins, minerals, amino acids, fats all come from? They were created through mitosis (cell replication), because no extra matter is coming in from the outside and this is what our body does all the time.

No food introduced into our bodies ever incorporates itself into the matrix of our cells, it only borrows nutrients for a short time by the body to help keep it stronger and provide such things as calories, salts, fats & hormones. Food should be consumed for just that reason, food as nourishment with the highest content of what our bodies need. This makes over eating a thing of the past. Nutrient rich food make one feel full very quickly.

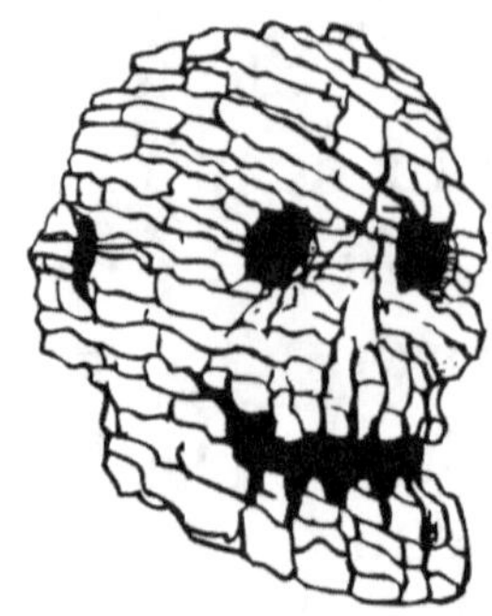

CALCIFICATION

There's a lot more to our bones overall health & strength than just calcium. Vitamins, minerals, sunlight, weight bearing exercise, to your posture, and even the way you sleep all have a truly profound impact. It is known in health and medical communities that too much calcium may cause cellular necrosis (cellular death). That is why pharmaceutical companies developed calcium channel blockers, to make sure the cells within the body do not get too much calcium at once. The ratio of calcium and magnesium found in plants are in perfect proportion to what our body needs. In animal & dairy, it is always way too high in calcium and very low in magnesium and very acidic, setting the body into a catabolic state, where it draws upon itself to maintain homeostasis.

Almost all of the calcium in the body is stored in bone. The rest is found in the blood. Excess calcium may be stored improperly in the bones, and may show up as arthritis.

By the age of 35 bone has finally stopped growing and you will only be at a loss after this stage if your diet is poor. This is why the three common forms of osteoarthritis and osteoporosis are never reversed, as the body cannot build more bone after a certain age, only slows or stops the progression.

Most doctors and even naturopaths, say that it's good to supplement with calcium, but they never tell you what kind or how much or when to take it. They may even neglect to perform such vital tests as coronary calcium score. If left neglected, while consuming high amounts of calcium can lead to a heart attack – a cause more common than elevated cholesterol levels! A coronary calcium score of zero indicates that there was no detectable calcium in your coronary arteries. Get a score of 80 and most doctors will consider not helping you as a patient.

Forms of Calcium

There are so many varieties of calcium that one should research, but what is the best? Low grade calcium carbonate and other such forms are weak in their ability to absorb, but still can help if one is very low. The best source is obviously "food derived" or "whole food" supplementation. I push people to these varieties rather than inorganic forms of calcium that the body is in danger of storing and really has a much harder time processing & absorbing. Calcium carbonate sources are usually oyster shells & can contain, dolomite, borine, nickel & lead.

Coral calcium is a ground-up fossilized animal that is hard for the body to assimilate and utilize. It can also contain unwanted trace elements, such as cadmium, uranium, and mercury.

The best way to assure bone health is to cut down the intake of protein. You may have heard that the acid-alkaline balance is the key factor, but this is secondary for bone health. Becoming alkaline is one of the absolute most important things one must strive for, but as far as bone health is concerned the restriction of high protein diets should be taken into consideration first, let me tell you why.

The acid alkaline balance is like your bodies temperature, if it varies off a few degrees above or below 98.6 degrees you can get very ill. The same applies to the bodies pH(Parts hydrogen) If it gets too far below 7.4 or above, the body compensates in a catabolic reaction, rather than making the body ill or feeling symptoms of sickness. It simply just starts to cannibalize itself to maintain homeostasis. Even though the body might be getting flooded with acid material all the time, the end result of this is going to be the body weakening itself of cell salts, immunity and cause great inflammation.

Almost all of the calcium in the body is stored in bone & cells. The rest is found in the blood. Normally the level of calcium in the blood is carefully controlled by the body. When blood calcium levels get low (hypocalcemia), the bones release calcium to bring it back to a good blood level. When blood calcium levels get high (hypercalcemia), the extra calcium is stored in the bones or passed out of the body in urine and stool. The amount of calcium in the body depends on the amount of calcium in your diet or supplementation, Vitamin D that your intestines absorb, phosphate levels in the body and also hormones.

Calcium Needs Acid

Calcium needs acid for proper assimilation. Without the proper strength acids, calcium is does not get dissolved and cannot be absorbed. Hydrochloric Acid (HA) is a vital acid in the stomach that helps us digest food, but as we eat poorly we often times we cannot produce enough hydrochloric acid. This is one reason that calcium and honey work so well with one another as honey has a lower pH and helps assist calcium absorption.

Sustainable and humanely gathered deer antler velvet taken with combination of iron-rich foods (i.e. molasses, Yacon syrup, prunes, pumpkin seeds, green hulls of black walnut) is found to be a powerful combo. Deer antler velvet helps the body to produce stem cells and iron is stored by the body in bone marrow. Iron is a very important mineral cannot get absorbed or utilized properly when its levels drop to low and then one can have a deficiency for life!

Skip the Calcium Fortification

DANGER: Skip all "enriched" or calcium "fortified" foods like yogurt, orange juice, soy milk etc. Manufacturers add calcium phosphate or tricalcium phosphate, which directly accounts for the high states of osteoarthritis, heart attacks & other bone related problems.

Limit or exclude cow milk all together, as this is liquid protein and every scientist knows that protein inhibits calcium absorption. This is what causes Irritable Bowel Syndrome (IBS), and over four million American women have this disorder. Denmark, Norway Holland & Sweden are the highest consumers of milk in the world. Guess which countries have the highest rate of osteoarthritis, osteoporosis & crippling bone disease? That's right: Denmark, Norway, Holland and Sweden.

(Fun fact: 60% of all cows in America have the leukemia virus, 80% have para-tuberculosis.)

There are over four thousand mammals and a half a million hormones but only one hormone in all of nature matches human, and that's a hormone found in cow's milk, and it the most powerful hormone in our body. You need these kinds of hormones when you are a baby, not so much when you are an adult. Milk has a hormone that makes breast cancer grow once you have it. Milk is composed of 80% casein and that's the same glue they use to put the label on the container of milk they sell. Essentially drinking 80% protein from casein is drinking mucus.

Sources for Calcium

The best food sources in the world for calcium are listed below.

- Nuts and Seeds: sesame, tahini, hemp, almonds, sunflower, pine nuts, walnuts, pecans, chia, flax, macadamia, brazil nuts, pumpkin seeds.

- Greens: kale, arugula, purslane, cabbage, mustard greens, broccoli, bok choy, chicory greens, turnip greens, borage, parsley watercress, cilantro, dandelion, lettuce, radishes, cauliflower, asparagus, artichoke, zucchini, okra, celery, mushrooms, aloe vera & collard greens.

- Seaweeds: kelp, nori, dulse, wakami, miso.

- Fruit: all berries, currants, grapes, tangerines, lemon, lime, cucumbers, cauliflower, avocado, onion, radish, currants, cherries, peaches, pears, pineapple, prunes, plums.

- Sprouts: alfalfa, broccoli & Brussels are extremely high in calcium

- Fermented foods: sauerkraut, kim chi, rejuvulack, are all wonderful for intestinal flora

- Bee pollen is amazing as it actually fights the virus that causes arthritis and honey helps to pull calcium into the bones and is a great food for our intestinal flora.

Aloe vera is part of the garlic family and it is very high in sulfur and is a powerful aid against arthritis. Aloe increases mineral absorption, and protein digestion. It contains over 200 compounds that aid the entire body and bile occlusion.

As we continue to witness and increase in major physical health disorders, science will be pointing the finger to calcification. Systemic disorders such as kidney stones, heart disease, prostate and breast cancer, even bone spurs will all have the same thing in common, calcification. Unfortunately I see our medical system only building more symptom-suppressing drugs as they focus their attention on pharmaceuticals. Yet diet has perhaps the greatest effect on the cause of all ailments, and health.

Try to obtain small amounts of calcium throughout the day, because calcium is absorbed in parts, rather than in one huge dose. Same with protein, the body can only assimilate some 25 grams at a single time, so more than that dosage is a waste of money. Giving a one-time shot of 1000mg is often times more burdensome for the system. Rather I tend to push people to 250mg four times a day if they are really needed to boost their calcium levels. Keep in mind calcium is best absorbed earlier in the day and magnesium more at night, as calcium tightens, magnesium relaxes. So it makes sense to take magnesium at night to help one relax and rest before bed and use calcium to wake up the system in the morning.

For someone with heart problems, gallbladder, kidney or other calcification problems, one really needs a lot less calcium in their diet and should especially watch for calcium phosphate added to foods. And it is added to almost everything. Some foods are also considered high oxalate and thus care and concern should be taken into consideration when under prior stress from stones or heart problems. Most all stones tested are made worse from calcium oxalate. Calcium oxalate is a chemical compound that forms needle-shaped crystals. Calcium oxalate crystals in the urine are the most common constituent of human kidney stones and calcium oxalate crystal formation is also one of the toxic effects of ethylene glycol poisoning.

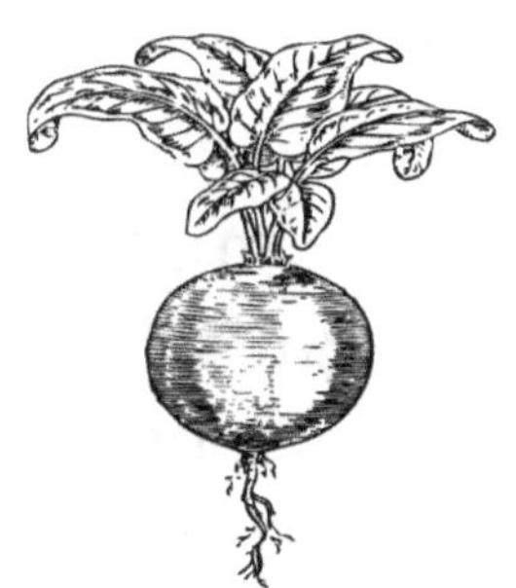

Calcium and Oxalic Acid

Oxalic acid, which is found in spinach, rhubarb, chard, agave and beet greens, peppers, tobacco, eggplant all bind with the calcium in themselves and reduces its absorption. These foods should not be considered good sources of calcium. Calcium in other green vegetables, like the ones listed above are absorbed better and can be eaten as long as long as one does not have kidney stones or other calcification problems.

Silica

Osteoporosis, basically means bones that are hollow, and my next area of study was finding as to how and why this happens.

New research by Dr. Louis Kervran on calcium assimilation concluded that animals do not eat calcium, yet they produce calcium in their bodies. He discovered that animals eat foods rich in minerals that actually biologically transmutate into other minerals required by the animals for metabolic processes. Since bone grows and replaces itself often, Dr. Kervran showed how organic plant-derived silica transmuted in the body to aid in bone production and strengthening.

A cow produces two to three gallons of calcium rich milk every day, yet the cow's diet is low in calcium. Grasses are approximately .001% calcium. The truth is that animals naturally produce up to twenty times more calcium than they ingest. Studies have proven that animals that eat silica-rich foods produce calcium as a terminal waste product.

In my humble opinion plant-derived silica is the best natural treatment for osteoporosis and calcium deficiency diseases. Many physicians have discovered that plant-derived silica, NOT calcium, has been shown to dramatically heal fractures and increase bone density and bone strength. Higher calcium intake is not the answer.

Most people don't know that too much calcium depletes the body of magnesium, and it's vital to have extra magnesium when you raise levels of calcium. Ideally I believe it's best to ingest Sulphur-bearing foods such as onions, garlic, aloe vera, noni, durian, and the supplement MethylSulfonylMethane (MSM), and silica such as Bio-Sil (has high absorption rate), bamboo, horsetail or cucumber, and a high grade magnesium citrate supplement to help move calcium to and from the cells as needed.

My additional protocol for Bone building is strontium supplementation, boron, Vitamin D3 (food derived calcium only and levels kept low!), and foods such as spirulina, greens, nuts and seeds, seaweeds, grasses, honey and pollen.

Never ever take steroids as they weaken bones and ligaments and tendons. An overactive parathyroid gland, hyperthyroidism, diabetes, anorexia, and chronic kidney failure also cause the bones to weaken.

WARNING: Vitamin D is essential for healthy teeth and bones. Our bodies can make Vitamin D from exposure to the sun, but this process turns off once our bodies have enough of the vitamin. However, when vitamin D is consumed as a supplement, there is no shut-off mechanism and an overdose can lead to abnormal calcium metabolism with symptoms such as nausea, constipation, weakness and bone pain. An excessive ingestion of Vitamin D usually occurs as a result of supplement overdose.

Test your calcium levels this way.

- To see if your disease symptoms may be caused by a very low calcium level in the blood, also known as hypocalcemia, notice is you have such symptoms like muscle cramps and twitching, repetitive muscle spasms, tingling in the fingers and around the mouth, muscle spasms, confusion, or depression, seizures and, possibly, cardiac arrhythmias.

- To see if your symptoms may be caused by a very high calcium level in the blood, also known as hypercalcemia, notice if you have such symptoms like muscle weakness, decreased muscle tone, lethargy, lack of energy, anorexia, not wanting to eat, nausea and vomiting, dehydration, constipation, polydipsia, and polyuria or urinating a lot, belly pain, or bone pain.

When calcium levels are greater than 13 mg/dL problems such as calcification in kidneys, gallbladder, skin, vessels, lungs, heart, and stomach occurs and renal (kidney) weakness may develop, especially if blood phosphate levels are normal or elevated due to impaired kidney function. Severe hypercalcemia may produce cardiac arrhythmias and worse and requires immediate intervention.

Strontium

Strontium is a common element which is naturally found in your bones. Strontium is also found in the soil and foods. As an alkaline earth element, strontium is similar to calcium in its ability to be absorbed in the gut, incorporated in bone, and eliminated through the kidneys. It is well-tolerated and believed to be completely safe.

Strontium combined with ranelic acid is used with great results increasing bone density by 12% on average. However strontium ranelate is registered as a prescription drug in Europe and many countries worldwide. It needs to be prescribed by a doctor, delivered by a pharmacist, and requires strict medical supervision. Currently, it is not available in Canada or the United States.

Nano Bacteria

In 1988 Finnish biochemist Olavi Kajander accidentally discovered mysterious particles that could potentially be responsible for sometimes fatal illnesses. These particles, a hundred times smaller than bacteria, seem to thrive inside dying cells. The Mayo Clinic has since supported many of the original findings on Nano bacteria; that they can self-replicate and cause calcification-related diseases. And calcification from Nano bacteria can triple in number in six hours on a diet consisting of cooked and dead microwaved foods.

My answer to this as of present is that all calcification-related issues such as heart attacks, gallbladder & kidney stones, bladder, osteoarthritis, and all age related disease are rooted from these Nano bacteria. In the zero-gravity of space, these bacteria grow five times as fast. Most stones essentially are formed from excessive starch consumption, but one would need the presence of Nano bacteria to calcify these indigestible proteins that lay stagnant in the gallbladder to make the situation worse. Bile occlusion needs to be removed and the liver needs to be working properly for one to turn calcification around and take action against this hidden enemy.

These bacteria build their shells with heavy metals floating around in the system, so assault them by fasting on high silica vegetable juices for two weeks while taking NCD Zeolites. After their shell is destroyed which could take a few months you need to destroy the bacteria which is best done by herbs. One of the most powerful and cheap ways is turmeric and garlic! These seem to fry these little bacteria and boost your immune system at the same time. A rare, but more powerful herb than garlic, is Chanca Piedra which literally means "stone breaker" due to its ability to break up calcium phosphate crystals (bad calcium). This super herb's historical use in achieving excellent gall bladder and kidney health is sizeable and well-studied. I also believe that the venom of bees also kills this bacteria.

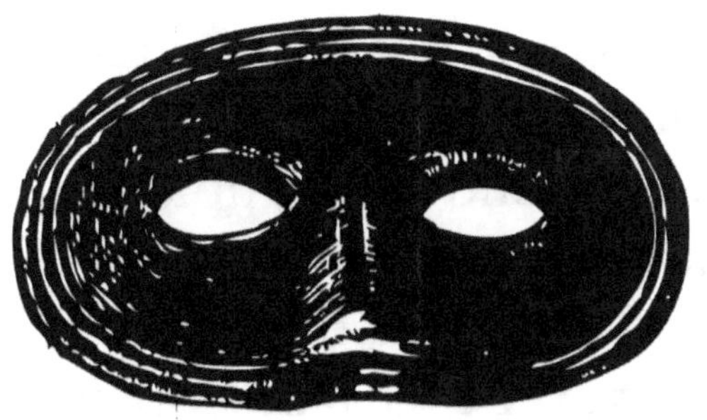

EYE HEALTH

The eyes are amazing and if you have ever closed them and walked around the house for even just a few minutes, you will realize how blessed you truly are for having this sense. Most people unfortunately are losing this amazing sense and now have to rely on glasses, contacts, or surgery to see. This is not what we were intended to have happen to us, and I believe that nutrition plays a vital role in eye health. Most people know about beta-carotene (Vitamin A) being good for the eyes and how carrots contain it. But that is all they know. Watermelon even contains high amounts of lutein and Vitamin A to strengthen eyesight. Some people know that cooked tomatoes contain lycopene, but raw blended tomatoes actually contain more than their cooked counterpart.

I find most people get more than enough vitamin A in their diet however and I actually do not recommend this supplement very often. Vitamin A is stored somewhat by the body and releases it as it needs it throughout the day. However this is only if you are consuming whole vegetables. Once a vegetable has been juiced its vitamin A content immediately enters into the blood stream and can't be stored properly. This is harsh on the liver and often makes us have vitamin toxicity. Ever seen someone who drinks lots of carrot juice? They actually change color, often times looking as orange as a carrot! This is because of the vitamin A not being able to be stored by the body but rather it is released all at once causing a huge burden on the entire system, forcing the body to attempt to eliminate the excess through the skin and urine.

I would rather prefer people reach towards a powerful vision-protecting anti-oxidant known as astaxanthin that is ten times stronger than all other antioxidants on the market. Also try to obtain your lycopene through flower petals or red berries because it is chemically bound to various types of fatty acids then. In these cases it is said that lutein is esterified and is commonly known as lutein ester. Lutein can be found predominantly from extracts of marigold flower extract, goji berries, squash, and bell peppers (red, orange and yellow).

Keep in mind that eye disorders are linked to fungus. Killing fungus and restoring the liver is key for bringing vitality back to eye health. Everything else is just secondary, so first fix the problem and then move on to beneficial additions to strengthen the eye.

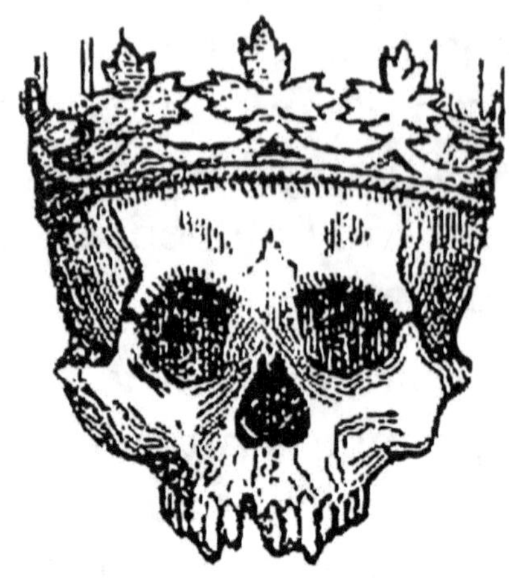

CANCER

Today's number one killer of children under the age of fifteen is cancer. According to the American Cancer Society estimated deaths from cancer in 2008 in the US is 565,650 adults. This number does not include children! The types of cancer that are most prevalent today are lung and bronchus. These cancers have outpaced cancer deaths with colon, prostate, stomach, breast and uterus. Since 1945 lung cancer has soared above all the rest. 22% of all deaths today are from cancer. The only disease more deadly in adults in America is heart disease, at 652,000 deaths.

My opinion is that the air we breathe today is the worst it has ever been in history. We have pollution everywhere and even polar bear cubs in Antarctica are found to have toxins in their blood. Without fresh air we won't last long as a species, we must take action now. Not only by the foods we eat, but a conscious lifestyle change that has concern for the future of our planet and our future generations.

My mother had stage three breast cancer when I was ten years old; she underwent chemotherapy and radiation therapy along with many surgeries to remove the tumors. After years of treatments she finally got over it, but ended up with lots of scars, and lost all of her hair. While this allopathic method worked for my mother I believe that these treatments are often times worse than the disease itself. It shuts off immunity, weakens the system and intestinal flora, damages all cells in the body (not just cancer cells) and worse than all it causes malnutrition.

Chemotherapy and radiation make one feel nauseated, dizzy, and lose your appetite. My mom hated the taste of everything! She could only taste metal in her mouth and found that only the highly sugary Chocolate Yoo-Hoo tasted good. Since one loses overall appetite while undergoing treatment, the body is starving for nutrients and statistics show that 40% of all cancer patients actually die from malnutrition!

The long term effects of medical treatments for cancer show many adverse side effects. I always advise moving towards a natural cure before considering harsh surgical pharmaceutical treatments. Being told you have cancer is obviously very scary. It's like being told you have a short time to live.

What doctors don't really recognize is that all cancer is caused by an intestinal blood parasite known in blood microscopy as a fluke. A holistic blood specialist can show you with a dark field microscope, cancer crystals in almost anyone's blood. What is bad however is when cancer builds to strong of a protein layer around it and the immune system can't differentiate between blood cells and cancer anymore. Then the cancer cells multiply faster than the body can fix itself. To dissolve this protein layer, new studies are looking at using unripe papaya skins which contain an enzyme papain that dissolves excess protein. When used in conjunction with the plant based enzyme protease it's even more effective.

In the next section I will list a few different protocols for fixing various forms of cancer, all through the gifts that our Heavenly Creator has given us through Mother Earth.

Chlorine Dioxide

Natural products generally cannot induce enough oxidative stress in cancer cells to actually kill them. Sodium chlorite, activated by vinegar to produce chloride dioxide, could be the oxidative agent that we have been looking for. It sounds too good to be true, but the science is sound.

In brief, sodium chlorite is treated with common white vinegar to produce chlorine dioxide, a powerful oxidant that is used in the purification of water, the bleaching of wood and cotton and other industrial uses. When generated, chlorine dioxide has a lifespan of only thirty minutes in the body, but this is enough to kill a host of different pathogens.

Walton C. Farr from West Virginia University has recorded how this simple compound successfully treated 37,000 people in Africa with malaria. Within 48 hours, this simple inexpensive compound killed 99% of all malaria pathogens. The author further maintains that this product may effectively kills HIV pathogens and many cancers, including pancreatic cancer.

Radiation

My friend Cassino died of a brain tumor at the age of 27, and when the cause was cancer the doctors had no idea what it was from. I took a step back and looked at it as environmental conditions, realizing that his job consisted of him being around electrical outlets & power lines daily. He worked for the telecommunications business, and started getting headaches while at work. He eventually became so disoriented that he fell down was unable to stand up and finally went to the hospital. He was told that he had a laceration of his cerebellum. This is what made him loose function of his coordination and he had to wear an eye patch while doing most activities. After one year of recovering and after surgery the cancer returned and finally took his life.

He was a physically strong and mentally sharp person. We trained martial arts together daily and worked out at the gym in our spare time. But even that was not enough to protect his body from the damage done by our environmental hazards of today. This is why we need to realize that the foods we eat are more than just nourishment for life, but are the key secrets to vitality, cleansing, free radical damage longevity & overall true health and vitality. We truly are what we eat!

Are you around computers a lot, or in the telecommunications business? Let's look at the foods that help the body around such burden of radiation: seaweeds, sunflower seeds & apples. These foods help the body when around such radiation because they fill the cells with pectin, so when radioactive pectin comes into contact with cells they are already full. Thus, food can protect cells against absorption of the dangerous radiation from powerlines, MRI, etc.

Make sure you read my chapter, "Raw Matt versus Cancer."

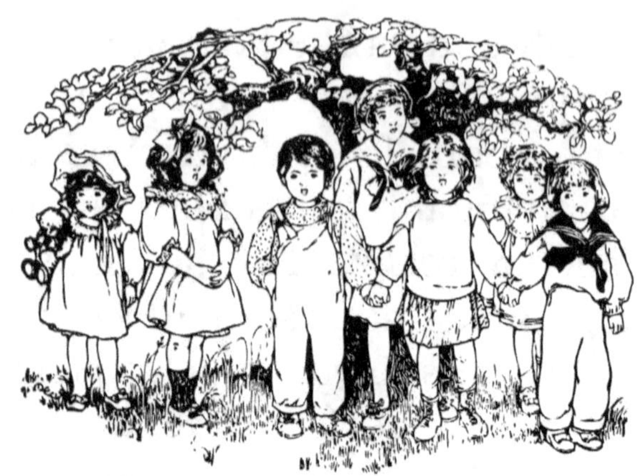

RAISED RAW?

Would a child benefit being raised on a raw vegan diet? Health wise yes, but socially, probably not. Imagine going to a public school, where everyone around you is eating all of the time. Kids live to eat, they live on junk food. If all adults died tomorrow, kids would be dead in weeks because they would raid the candy stores and live off pure sugar.

In my opinion, the only way to raise a kid raw would be home schooling. This may be best, because really, what life lessons do you learn in public school anyway? How to not get your ass kicked for your lunch money is about it. The only detriment to home schooling is the lack of social interaction with other kids. You can counteract this by getting them involved in sports, martial arts, or other activities where they will meet other kids and learn how to interact with them.

I have yet to see any kids being raised on a hundred percent raw vegan diet, but I absolutely believe it can be done. I personally wish I had been raised that way, but at least I know better now. One day we will start seeing kids being raised this way. And I bet you now that you will be seeing some healthy kids.

Most people in today's world see how bad and toxic it is becoming, but few are actually willing to step up the plate and DO something about it. We all point fingers at and complain about the oil companies and think that is enough. We need to be much more conscious than ever before, making better decisions daily. Make sure your kids get what they need to grow - this is of the utmost importance, and information leads to confidence.

Kids metabolisms are very fast and they burn off calories faster than an adult. Because the brain is by far the most energy demanding organ of the body, kids need optimal fuel so they don't mentally burn out. As adults we become exhausted when we must concentrate for long periods of time. As where kids can mentally learn much better because they take longer to fatigue. Since their bodies work so much more efficiently than ours do and they are more 'open systems,' they are also much more susceptible to pathogens, carcinogens, and toxic chemicals than we are as adults. This is why cancer is the number one killer among children. Their skin is more affected by hormones than adults are also; this is the reason for such bad acne. Bad food, plus unbalanced hormones throws the body off.

Kids are hit from every angle, they see on TV Ronald McDonald touting fatty hamburgers with kids all around him in a playhouse, and well, they want to be doing that just like the kids on TV. They don't understand about media or corporate manipulation going on. Why do you think all the cereals at the grocery stores with cartoons and pictures on them are all kids' height? Those companies pay a lot for those shelves to entice kids to grab those cereal boxes and they are nothing but cardboard sugar laden crap. It's sad that people only care about money and that innocent people have to suffer for it.

Ignorance is not bliss. But that's where being conscious and awake matters in life. That is the reason for this book. And that is why all this information has been compiled here for you. It's to inform you about everything that seems trivial or overlooked in life, but really does matter. We are all a part of it. There are many wolves among us and like wolves, they prey on the weak and lame. Be powerful and dominant and healthy!

Kids need to be outside playing in the sun, not inside watching Sponge Bob and other mindless garbage, eating ice cream and playing video games all day long. These things don't stimulate the brain to grow at all, they waste time. Kids need to physically be active, and the sun helps them mellow out as it gives the brain proper melatonin levels. When a kid sits in front of a TV all day long, their body has built up stored energy. Now they can't or don't want to go to sleep, because they sat on their asses all day long. Now school is just that much harder to concentrate in, because they have just too much energy to sit still.

So then in comes the doctor to say, "Your Kids have ADHD," and throw their asses on drugs. Now the poor kid, not having anything but natural child energy, is being punished for having what? Energy? See the problem? It's all a repetitive cycle. Today over 8 million kids are on methylphenidate, (sold under trade names like 'Ritalin,') a central nervous system (CNS) stimulant? Or amphetamine (sold under the trade name, Adderall) another stimulant?

UNACCEPTIBLE!

Natural foods, sunlight, physical activity and friendship are all part of what a child needs to do daily. Yeah, it's important to study, but for the mind to work, the body must be healthy. A child's minds is so scattered, any parent can tell you that one minute they want to watch a movie and then one minute later they want to go skate or play games or you name it. And all this excess sugar and hormone-filled foods really make it tough for kids. This is where it's up to the parents to make the right decisions in buying healthy organic foods and cutting the crap out of their kids' diets.

Some of the best foods for children are hemp seeds, bee products (honey, pollen, propolis & royal jelly) – just make sure not to give any of these to children under one year of age. These all have powerful enzyme content, vitamins, minerals and nutrients a body craves. Pollen is the most easily digested protein there is. It's a free form amino acid complex, not a chain of protein the body has to break down to amino acids. Thus, the body has no processing to do and the nutrition immediately becomes absorbed. Hemp seeds contain high amounts of omega 3, 6, 9 & 18 EFAs and are great for a growing brain. Because hemp seeds are the only seeds that do not contain enzyme inhibitors, they are easy to use without sprouting or soaking. Be sure to use the whole hulled hemp seed and not the oil, as the oil is too concentrated and can throw hormones off-balance is used in excess.

Rice Bran Solubles

Rice Bran Solubles (RBS) contain alpha lipoic acid which helps control blood sugar, and in itself is a powerful antioxidant. RBS is my top supplement I recommend; it contains glutathione peroxidase (a metabolic enzyme) that is used by the body to perform all sorts of actions. The Vitamin E in RBS is a THOUSAND time stronger than any antioxidant found in any other nut or seed. The vitamin E tocotrinals found in RBS protect the brain from nitrogenous (organic compounds like ammonia) free radical scavengers. Because our brain and cells are made of fat, the vitamin E in RBS protects not just cell membranes but the cells in the brain as well. It should be noted that rice naturally accumulates arsenic from the soil, so just like everything else, use your natural medicines in moderation.

Fruit contains hydrating organic liquids that fuel the body through carbohydrates, but do not causing an increase in insulin so the kid never gets a sugar rush like candy does. Unlike nuts and seeds, fruit doesn't contain enzyme inhibitors that give the body a hard time processing. So fruit is easy to digest. Children love sweets, and after mothers milk, put them on is a nice blended fresh fruit juice. Greens are best juiced, but fruit are better blended, as this holds the fiber and keeps the GI of the food much lower. And kids love melons (cantaloupe and honeydew). Blend the meat of them up and watch them drink away!

Next Generation

My prediction for our next generation being raised in the most polluted, toxic environment ever in human history, is still good. I believe that because of all the astounding research and scientific evidence and the access to obtain it easily, that their lives can be long and healthy.

Right now over 64% of the children in America are obese, but this is simply their parents' fault. When these kids become older they will hopefully take responsibility for their own health and when they see that diet affects everything. I hope they will see how foods affect their mental and physical well-being and see the light themselves.

Every year we get better and better with technologies, science, applications, and learning. The most basic of all of these and easiest for ANY of us to change is our diet. This is why most of my attention has been on this one aspect.

You can't start to run if you never learned to walk. You must learn the basics first. I urge you to take the fear out of your minds and apply this simple philosophy for yourselves and family that we truly are what you eat, think and believe. And nothing is stronger than your own mind.

TECHNOLOGIES

*"Nothing will benefit human health
and increase chances for survival of life
on Earth as much as the evolution
to a vegetarian diet."*

Albert Einstein

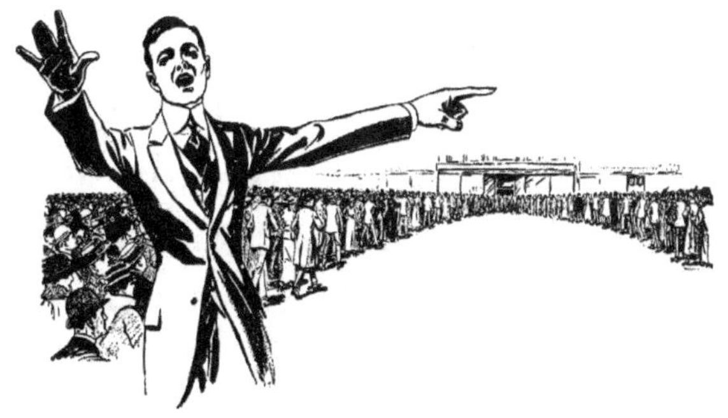

THERAPEUTIC MODALITIES

Hydrotherapy

Hydrotherapy was designed and practiced in India and then in Rome. Hydrotherapy today is not practiced nearly enough. This simple procedure can rid someone of the flu, or even prevent it if done daily as a preventative. Teaching your body to get accustomed to cold water hydrotherapy can help you build strength against cold weather. Cold water can make blood vessels in your skin clamp down faster so you lose less warmth in cold exposure. If someone has the flu, set them in a bath of ice water for three minutes and then getting out and massage until they are warm again and repeat. You may also alternate hot and cold water in a shower for thirty to sixty seconds at each temperature. These therapies makes cells vibrate higher, blood flow faster and release toxins at a faster rate, making them stronger at knocking out viruses. More technically, ice cold water increases interleukin-4 and gamma interferon, which are two of our body's virus-fighting cytokines.

Herbal Remedies

Herbs have been used for hundreds if not thousands of years in healing. I am particularly fond of herbs as natural remedies. However, because they are best consumed in their whole natural state, they are not readily prescribed by traditional doctors. They are overlooked because of the pharmaceutical industry's hold on how people view medical treatment and remedies. The reason you have not nor will ever hear about these natural remedies is because that unless someone can put a patent on something, there is otherwise no money to be made. This makes herbs such as graviola, bloodroot, turmeric and shilijit largely unpublished in medical journals, because they cannot synthesize the active constituents in the herb to put a patent on it and make millions of dollars. Being able to just take the herb and become well would make them zero dollars.

However keep in mind that some people have reactions to certain herbs. Thus, I advise using caution the first time you take anything. I treat nature with respect and never neglect that some herbs can really cause harm. Here is the protocol that I use when trying all new forms of food.

When everyone is partaking in nature hikes, backpacking, forging, or anything that can introduce a new substance to your diet, try this. Let's say for instance you are trying a fruit for the first time. Puncture the fruit, open it with your nail, and rub it on a small patch of skin. If there is no reaction after ten to fifteen minutes, rub the juice on your mouth & lips.

After about five minutes without any reaction take a small bite and chew it up and spit it out. After five more minutes without a reaction you can pretty much conclude you do not have an allergic skin reaction to the food. Next consume some of the fruit and wait about ten minutes. This will be your factor in determining if the food is palatable for further consumption. I realize this process is time consuming, but getting sick or having a worse reaction is much more detrimental. This technique I have used for many things and it has yet to fail me, even when living in the jungles of Kauai.

After you have found out you are not allergic to a certain herb, healing with herbs is probably one of my favorite and most simple ways to purge the system of things like parasites, metals, imbalances & toxins in general. Generations before us took advantage of herbalism for thousands of years before pharmaceutical solutions became available. So to me that's more of a tried and trusted way to go about healing, where little guesswork needs to get done. The side effects and long term health effects aren't just mere guess work (like today's over the counter drugs approach). Today 25% of all pharmaceuticals are still herb based! You're just not getting them in their intended true whole form.

Powerful Substances

Cutting edge research is going on all the time looking at nutritional solutions to common ailments. There have been several powerful substances that have been shown to help the body remedy itself, like Vitamin B17, a powerful T-cell builder found in apricot seeds, red clover and wheat grass. The supplement known as rice bran solubles contains antimutagenic compounds. Inositol, a B vitamin, IP6, polyphenols, tocotrienols, and other antioxidants are proving to be very powerful anti-carcinogens. Zeolites, which I have already mentioned, have a lot of research showing its effectiveness in healing.

Gaviola, an amazing tree is found in the Amazon rainforest is showing to have incredible promise in the treatment of cancer. It has been used for its ability to kill parasites, but was later found to attack cancer cells while leaving normal cells unharmed.

Turmeric

And let's not forget trusty ole turmeric. Turmeric is anti-inflammatory and also protects the liver which detoxifies the body, but it also has been proven effective at destroying certain types of cancer cells. The researchers at the University of Texas M.D. Anderson Cancer Center conducted a study that showed when curcumin from turmeric was introduced into cell cultures containing multiple melanoma, it stopped the cancer cells from reproducing and those that were left died!

These are all basic herbs that anyone in America can obtain. For instance cayenne pepper increases body circulation. Cumin is great for an anti-tumor protectant. Garlic is a powerful cleanser, and used as an anti-cancer and immune boosting herb. These herbs can be very powerful and I never recommend any of them daily for over a four month period. They should be used for special healing, not daily upkeep. When you have something that WORKS as well as herbs do, they push the immune system to a very high status causing what is known today as auto-immunity. We do not need our immune system this high constantly, as it is more hindering than beneficial in the long run.

Juicing

Juice, in terms of vegetable juice, is one of the best ways one can rejuvenate the entire body. I believe limiting juice to one or two at most a day at best, because one can really over consume if you juice more than this. However as far as clean up goes, nothing is faster and easier on the digestive track. I suggest to juice predominantly vegetables and small amounts of fruit, as the sugar content is greatly increased when fruit is juiced and fiber has been removed. When fruit is juiced it immediately enters into the bloodstream and can cause runaway blood sugar. Avoid fruit juices and fruit additions altogether if you are diabetic or sugar sensitive.

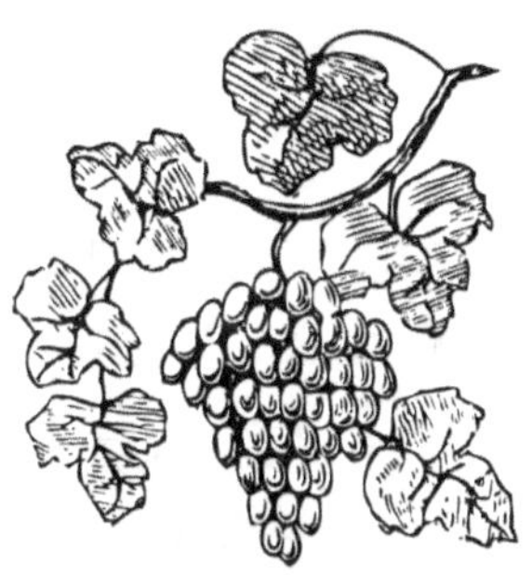

I tend to keep carrots and beets below ten percent of the liquid of vegetables in any juice because they also are high in sugar, and suggest a base predominantly either celery or cucumber. Great additions to any juice are parsley, chard, cabbage, dandelion, kale, cilantro, ginger or garlic. Adding lemon or lime keeps juice fresher longer if you plan on storing it.

Juice is the best breakfast one can have, as breakfast is the perfect time for re-hydration of cells in the body. Since the body naturally drops more acidic at night, fresh vegetable juice flushes the system with high alkaline material that energizes the system fast and thoroughly. Anyone looking for more energy throughout the day should try fresh cold pressed vegetable juice. At least in the beginning stages of a raw food diet, eventually you will get off vegetable juice and skip it all together. Vegetable juice is great for getting the body acclimated to start consuming vegetables on a regular basis.

After you've been eating better (hopefully mostly raw) for a while, I only recommend juicing when on a cleanse, such as a heavy metal cleanse, as you want to produce as much urine as possible during this time.

I mainly advocate soups and blended meals rather than juicing, as nutrients and fiber are often lost in the juicing process.

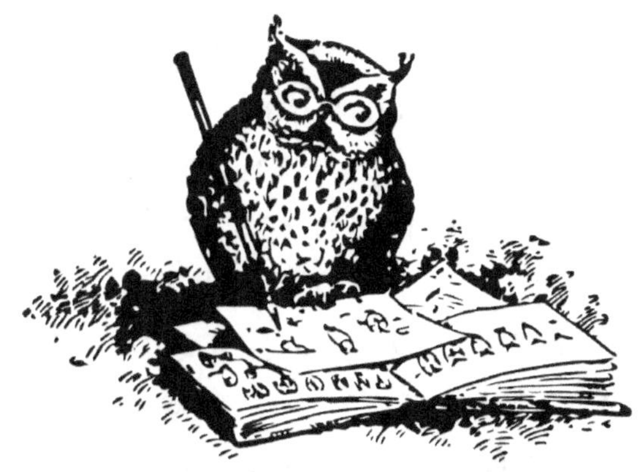

THE DE-STRESS EFFECT

What is amazing is that some diseases can arise from within, without cause of diet, but simply from stress. Such stress related diseases are leprosy, tuberculosis, salmonella, a typhoid-like (rod shaped) bacteria and flux. Stress increases cortisol release in our bodies and creates a whole host of issues, including weight gain, high blood pressure, skin disorders like acne and eczema, and the aforementioned serious ailments.

Counteract stress with a relaxed attitude, yoga, meditation, and a calm environment. If you are a perfectionist or a control freak, realize that you don't have to be perfect or be in control for things to turn out just fine. It will be much easier and much more relaxing for you to let things take their course. You WILL be okay and your life will turn out fine if the dog pees on the floor, or a grocery cart makes a little ding in your car door (unless it's a Lamborghini, then freak out all you want and hunt down the person who did it), or you're running five minutes late. These little things don't matter at all. Do yourself a huge favor and let them go.

Yoga and meditation are also great for re-wiring a stressed out nervous system or Type A personality. Just three thirty to sixty minute sessions per week at the local yoga studio will do wonders for your stress levels and help you manage your weight more easily. You can meditate anytime by simply taking several deep belly breaths for at least one minute, closing your eyes, smiling, and either saying mentally or out loud that you appreciate life, your body, your health and your God. Just take a moment to breathe in and be grateful.

It is also a good idea to take an hour or so to clear up any clutter or disorganization in your work or living space. Other cultures, such as the Japanese, are naturally inclined to be less stressed, which is attributed to their adherence to a system known as Feng Shui, which focuses on balancing energy in the home for optimum health and a positive life. Clutter subconsciously stresses us out, so dump the unnecessary crap in the garage. If you haven't looked at it or used it in several months or years, chances are you never will, so get rid of it. Simplify your life and feel the stress disappear.

Another suggestion is to get a few green houseplants. They filter the air and create a calming appearance. Even fresh flowers every so often are a great addition to the environment. Running water in the form of a little desk fountain is also awesome, as they help to generate negative ions that strip the air of toxins and elevate your mood. Whatever makes you happy to look at and calms you down, put it in your most commonly used space.

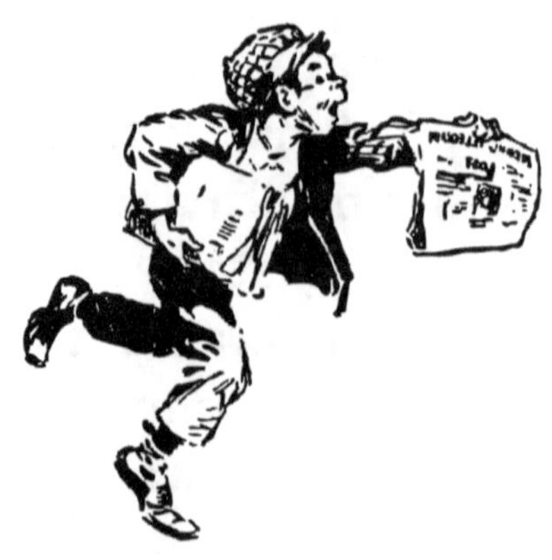

CLEANSING

Jumping right into cleansing or fasting straight off of the Standard American Diet (SAD) is not a good idea. Our fat is designed to hold toxins and release them slowly into the blood stream, so that we can detoxify them through either the stool, lymphatic system or skin and not feel sick. Ever wonder why some people often look sick when they shift to an all vegetarian, vegan or raw food diet too fast? If you try to "detox" (the dreaded word) too unnaturally fast, you are just asking for major trouble.

Exercise is one way of slowly cleansing the system out this, but it does not come close to being as powerful as a major dietary change. But some people have more body fat, which means more accumulated toxins. When these people loose fat too quickly, they release these toxins into their blood stream very fast. This makes one feel quite sick, and very moody. For me it was more mental chaos, because I was still constantly working out, I was able to sweat out most of the toxins without really knowing fully what was happening.

Colon Cleanse

Now most people do not have tons and tons of fecal matter like some of those nasty colon cleansing pictures you may have seen before. Regardless, the colon is a breeding ground for parasites, as it is a moist, damp habitat for these little bastards. Thankfully, the colon can be flushed pretty fast. If you have ever seen a camera view from inside the colon, it is actually pretty clean after a simple flush. It looks all pink and clean like the back of your throat.

Most detox centers recommend starting with a colon cleanse (but in my opinion the best cleanse to start with is a liver cleanse). I certainly agree and recommend getting a series of three to six colonics over a three to six week period to for a cleansing regimen. If you are overweight or suspect you have a high toxic overload due to your environmental conditions or dietary choices (i.e. a diet high in factory farmed meat, starch, processed foods, soda, etc.), opt for six colonics in a three to four week period. Give your body at least a three day rest between colonics. After doing this colon cleanse program and maintaining healthy diet, you can choose to maintain a quarterly detox protocol by doing a total of one to four colonics per year. Even an enema would suffice.

After a colon cleanse I would relax for a while. It's nice to give the body a break. If the body is always processing something or working hard to clean up debris, it will take its toll. Jumping from one cleanse to another will just make one sick or lose weight too quickly. And some people get addicted to cleansing which in itself to me appears to border on an unhealthy mental obsession. I recommend four months rest before starting a different cleanse. Just think to yourself, I will start my next detox or cleanse quarterly.

Do not get what is called a 'closed system' colonic. This is a process where the therapist puts a rather large tube in the patient's rectum, and the system forces water in and forces it back out. The size of the tube is a concern and can in some cases cause rectal or colon ruptures. And if the obstruction is larger than the width of the tube, it cannot pass. Instead look for a colon hydrotherapy center that offers an 'open system.' This is a relaxing process, involving a tube smaller than a pinkie finger, and over the course of 45-60 minutes, you are flushed with warm water and release when you are comfortable. This also exercises your colon, so if you suffer from chronic constipation or sluggish digestion, this will help get your intestinal system back in shape without relying on colonics or enemas.

Support Your Intestines

Support your intestinal tract during this time with three to four liters of filtered spring water, three to five servings of fresh fruits for fiber, and enzyme supplementation daily.

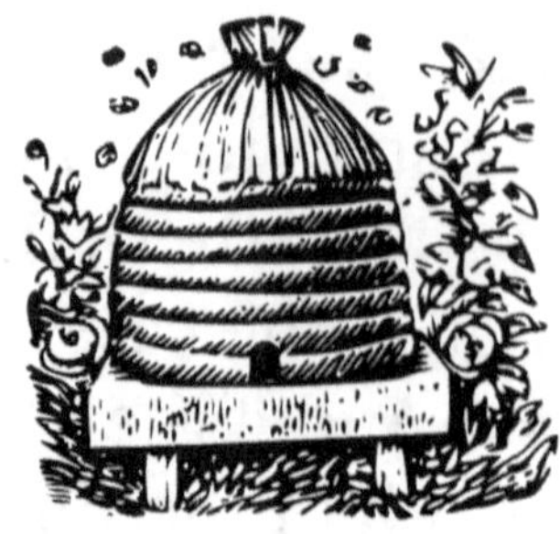

A great food to take is honey, as honey contains antioxidants that have been implicated in reducing the damage done to the colon in colitis related to inflammation. Fiber is obviously a good thing to take, but unfortunately it is just sold as simply fiber, such as psyllium, acacia, flax etc. Fiber acts like a broom to push congested material through the bowls, colon and intestines. Brown or heirloom varieties of rice make a good intestinal broom. Most cleanses work best when in conjunction with blended vegetable which are low in calories and high in fiber. Vegetable blending or steaming while on a colon cleanse is a great combo. Try celery, parsley, cabbage, cucumber, cilantro and ginger in different combinations. However, fiber alone without potassium is worthless, as potassium acts like a pump, contracting and relaxing the intestines to help fiber flush through your system more effectively.

Get your potassium from apple cider vinegar, blackstrap molasses, yams (cooked, preferably baked without oil in the oven), papaya, celery, cucumber, grapes, raisins, banana, and grapefruit. Vegetable juices are low in calories, high in a variety of nutrients, and encourage good gut flora.

Liver Cleanse

After the colonics, do a liver cleanse. The liver is by far the most important organ to cleanse and to remove bile occlusion. The liver and gallbladder are both flushed in the same manner. It will take a process of about two months to fully rid the body of stones that have accumulated. There are a few different ways of liver cleansing and I advocate the easiest kind of cleanse.

Start by strengthening the liver via a simple two week program of herbs and minerals and basic diet change, and use de-calcification techniques to remove calcified & non-calcified stones that have accumulated. As far as the diet is concerned, one should move toward more blended soups, liquids to let the liver get a break. The liver is the hottest organ of the body because it's always processing something. Moving towards a regimen of blended fruits and greens, in the form of soups and smoothies really adds much more vital nutrients than you might expect. Unlike juicing, which removes important fiber and nutrients, one can rejuvenate the liver enough to strengthen its ability to flush out stones.

Although the liver can process over eighty thousand pounds of food (that's over forty tons) in a lifetime, it is a good idea to give it a rest now and then. The liver, once clear of stones will dramatically improve your digestion. One can clear up eyesight, tooth pain, kidney problems, allergies, even shoulder, back and upper arm pain & a whole list of aliments unimagined just through a simple liver cleansing program.

It is the job of the liver to make bile, one to one and a half quarts in a day! The gallbladder is attached to the common bile duct and acts as a storage reservoir or garbage dump for the liver. The consumption of fat or protein triggers the gallbladder to squeeze itself empty after about twenty minutes, and the stored bile finishes its trip down the common bile duct to the intestine.

Today's food pyramid is completely full of starch. If the gallbladder & liver are working to digest cooked starch then the liver will release bile and enshroud these particles, and often times these particles get stored in these organs. This is what accumulates and slowly becomes calcified stones in time. Most people, even kids are littered with stones. What's really scary is that at the very center of each stone is found a clump of bacteria, according to scientists, suggesting a dead bit of parasite might have started the stone forming. Current research is pointing the finger at parasites and Nano bacteria that can never become dislodged on their own. Only by cleansing will these debris ever come loose, no matter how good your diet becomes.

Gallstones

Most people don't know that there are over half a dozen varieties of gallstones, most of which have cholesterol crystals in them. They can be black, red, white, green or tan colored. The green ones get their color from being coated with bile. Some even find fluke remains, (a parasite that lives in the liver). Some stones are composites of many smaller ones, showing that they regrouped in the bile ducts sometime after the last cleanse. Thus, I recommend doing six to fourteen flushes every week to get the liver back to its full capacity.

As the stones grow and become more numerous and calcified the pressure on the back of the liver causes it to produce less and less bile. Imagine that your garden hose had marbles in it. Much less water would flow, which in turn would decrease its ability to squirt out the marbles. With gallstones, much less cholesterol leaves the body, and cholesterol levels rise.

Gallstones, being porous, can pick up all sorts of bacteria, cysts, fungus, viruses and parasites that are passing through the liver. In this way "pools" of infection are formed, forever supplying the body with harmful bacteria. Even diluting all the food you eat.

o stomach infection, such as ulcers or intestinal bloating can ever be cured permanently without removing these stones from the liver, that is how important this cleanse is. Not even changing your diet in the strictest way will clear away these impediments, thus it's our job to dislodge these accumulated stones for good.

Liver and Gallbladder Cleanse

Gall bladder removal surgery (cholecystectomy) is one of the top surgeries performed in America today, and I'm sick and tired of the lies that pour out of our modern day health care facilities. They are nothing but unfocused distracted individuals, with poor intentions on understanding of true health. Our modern day medical program has failed us. Until we all open our eyes and look around to see that everyone is on some kind of medication will we begin to see that we, as a nation have lost our health.

This is a very important cleanse, because bile has to be flowing properly in order for food to flow through the intestinal track, allowing the colon to empty itself normally.

You may have heard of a "liver flush" protocol involving olive oil, Epsom salts, and castor oil packs. I have tried this cleanse many times and found that it is actually detrimental to the liver. The liver now has to process a massive quantity of fatty oil and it is a burden for the liver to have to do this. I have seen first-hand, laboratory results of the gallstones that come out after this cleanse, and they are, in fact, simply olive oil/epsom salt/bile mixtures. They are not gallstones. As a result, I no longer teach people how to do this flush and advocate an effective herbal cleanse for the liver.

Herbs such as chanca piedra (stone breaker), milk thistle seed, dandelion root, turmeric root (take with black pepper), and boldo leaf all assist in flushing the gallbladder and liver. Keep in mind that bitter herbs in general will stimulate bile flow and liver efficiency, so try to keep them in your daily diet.

When helping your liver and gallbladder clean out, drink water with fresh squeezed lemon in the morning and enjoy warm dandelion and milk thistle teas, as this also stimulates the liver. You may also drink warm chanca piedra tea – simply boil three cups of water and add one tablespoon of the herb and let it steep for about fifteen minutes.

The stronger you want your liver the more you let it rest, drinking warm teas are revitalizing to this organ. Cold is stimulating and causes the liver to contract, so avoid cold drinks and smoothies as much as possible.

Once your liver has begun to work without impediment of stones, it can again be able to take in sugar, not stress the body, and stop feeding Candida and the bile will be flowing. This is what neutralizes the acid in the stomach when food taken in, and assists the breakdown of fats and sugars.

Heavy Metals Cleanse

The heavy metal cleanse is the final cleanse, and should not be overlooked. The predominant heavy metals are mercury, led, cadmium & arsenic.

Recent research shows that heavy metals are food for parasites, immune destroyers, and cancer and they accumulate in the fat, blood and brain tissue over time. Heavy metals enter our bodies the same way parasites can, through drinking water, eating food, cooking with metal, inhalation, vapor, and even tattoos. I have learned that the hard way.

Depleted Uranium (DU) is found in thirty nine out of forty Americans! This neurotoxin is the reason so many children are being born without eyes and arms over in Iraq right now. Our military shell casings contain DU, and when guns are fired the vapor is almost instantly inhaled.

There are a few ways to cleanse heavy metals. EDTA chelates most, but leaves mercury behind and is a slower process and must be done intravenously, not orally. There have been actual studies done on humans to show that after one month of proper usage 99% of people taking zeolites were free of heavy metals. However, these kinds of products can be very expensive.

I like Natural Cellular Defense brand because all zeolites are naturally already full of heavy metals, but a chemist in a small pharmaceutical company in Ohio researched and purified them. He was given a patent #6,288,045 by the US government. He made the zeolites similar to distilled water, as it is simply stripped of all minerals. So when you ingest it, it attracts all heavy metals in your body toward IT and you simply urinate them out. Studies being done now are showing promising results with zeolites on autism and even cancer.

I have an extreme protocol for heavy metal chelation, but like most cleanses I like to just do them one time and do it right! Liquid fasting with zeolites is again the best. Taking sun chlorella powder or liquid is a great addition as it is high in minerals while you are fasting, and also has enzymes. I also recommend modifilan which is a brown seaweed derived from laminaria joponica (hoku kombu). It was designated as a leading remedy for the rehabilitation of the Chernobyl nuclear catastrophe victims. It helps to remove lead, mercury, uranium & strontium which EDTA often leaves behind. There is heavy metal research is currently supported by the National Science Foundation, the Department of Energy, Shell Global Solutions, Sandia National Laboratories and the American Chemical Society-Petroleum Research Fund. So I think we are onto something!

As a side note – there are some proponents of an advanced therapeutic method called Urine Therapy – which you can imagine part of what that involves. If you subscribe to this method, never ever do it when you are cleansing – especially a heavy metals cleanse, as the toxins are released through your urine.

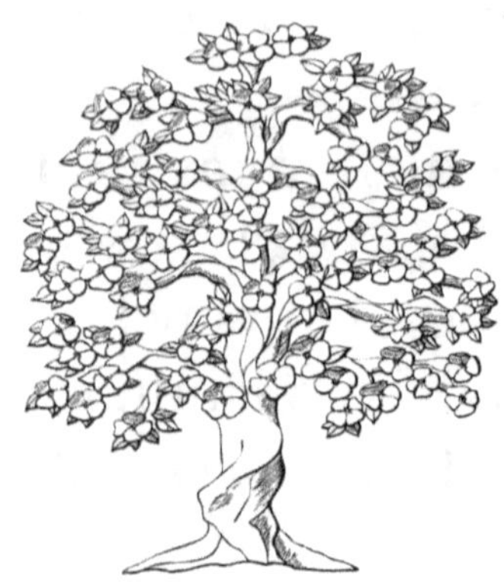

FIXING FUNGAL INFECTIONS

The number one thing for killing Candida is a probiotic called acidophilus. I follow probiotics with a ten day internal consumption of colloidal silver with grapefruit seed extract for one month. Goji berry juice and aloe vera are also powerful destroyers of fungus. Watch the glycemic index of the foods you ingest as everything you eat turns into sugar in the body and fungus needs sugar to survive. Keeping your foods low glycemic is key for success. Make sure you consider doing a liver flush also so that all bile occlusion is gone and proper assimilation can occur.

A great anti-fungal herbs that are as potent as the over-the-counter antifungal drugs includes tabebuia impetiginosa (pau d'arco bark) Pau d'arco taken with chaparral makes the strength 3 times stronger! Goldenseal root & Oregon grape root are also highly effective antiseptic and antibiotics. They contain a germ-killing compound called bebeerine that activates white blood cells to fight against infection. They help rid the body of many types of bacteria and fungi including those that cause Candida (yeast) infections, ringworm, viruses, and various parasites such as tapeworms and giardia. The usual dose is a third of a teaspoon with 1 glass of water, 3 times daily.

Note that just like pharmaceutical antibiotics, goldenseal and these other anti-fungal should not be taken over a long period of time because they can adversely affect healthy bacteria. You can compensate this by adding acidophilus to the diet.

Fasting

Fasts are done for many reasons such as spiritual, health, weight loss, or even necessity. Fasting can be one of the best things ever done for your health as this gives the body time to recover and do clean up. Fasting on nothing but water can be detrimental over time, because we have been eating wrong before the fast ever begins. And fasting improperly can cause problems to worsen if done wrong.

There are some simple steps to take before jumping into a fast more than a couple of days. It is not as important for a short one day fast, because ketosis will not set in with such a short fast. Ketosis is a starvation state in your body where the body runs off sugar for energy first, but soon after the liver starts to metabolize fats into fatty acids and ketones to give the body a source of energy.

Why do you think kids in Ethiopia die of starvation? Most of these kids get a bag of white rice once a week through Red Cross donation. Shouldn't that be giving them the nutrition they need? The answer to that may shock you. Most of those poor kids do not die from starvation.

The white rice they consume causes fungus in the body. Grains and other starches send a signal to the digestive track after consumption that a form of sugar needs to be processed. But because this food is without natural cell salts, has a high glycemic or glucose digestive enzymes, it causes great sweet & fat cravings. The rice also induces celiac disease and weakens their immune system further, making them more susceptible to peristalsis and disease.

Sadly 25% of these kids die from parasites, 65% disease, and 10% starvation. When tested, amazingly the kids in these third world countries were higher mineralized than our kids here in America! There are simple steps we could take that could teach people how to live in a way congruent with Mother Earth rather than have reliance on our grains.

I tell you this, because fasting is not dangerous or unnatural, nor do we need food every single day in order to live.

The simple process of stopping the high consumption of flesh foods would reduce resource, land and water usage, and cut down the massive greenhouse gases that pour out of animal farms, more than any other single tragedy going on right now. Reducing flesh consumption is the biggest step we could take towards helping everyone around the world. What's simply amazing to me is that not only would cutting meat out of the diet benefit our planet, resources, water, but it would allow us to feed most of the world. It's the most optimal for our long term health!

Flesh foods congeal blood, acidify the body, and burden the liver and most organs. Animal fats contain high levels of toxins and cholesterol. Most cows have leukemia and many other diseases and cancer. 100 years ago this was not the case, but today most animals and fish are farm raised under horrible conditions. The animals are filled contaminates we in turn ingest. As our body is a machine and it can work fine for a while but if you keep filling the gas tank with low grade fuel, eventually it catches up to you. So raw vegan…good for the planet and good for you. Duh!

Here are a couple ideas of ways to fast.

- If it's your first fast consider mixing spring water with unheated honey, turmeric juice, lemon or lime juice, and a pinch of Celtic sea salt. Consider consuming digestive enzymes every hour for the three days. This mixture is what will make the fast easy, because hunger is less likely than simply jumping into a water-only fast. This first timer fast really helps aid the body in removal of toxins and debris. By continuing to give the body "something to chew on," it doesn't allow the body to enter ketosis.

Blood Fast

Another fast I recommend is a blood cleanse, it's about a two week fast that encourages uptake of nutrients by the cell. What you need for this is

- Spring water

- Sun chlorella or spirulina, your choice

- Exogenous Ketone Supplements

- High doses of digestive enzymes.

This two week cleanse involves awaking to water with high potency plant based digestive enzymes. Every few hours consume small amounts of enzymes regardless if taken with anything else. About four times throughout your day you will be consuming either one tablespoon of spirulina or sun chlorella. It's best taken as tablet form and chewed well, but if you do not desire the taste simply swallow with water. Take the ketone alone in-between even water consumption.

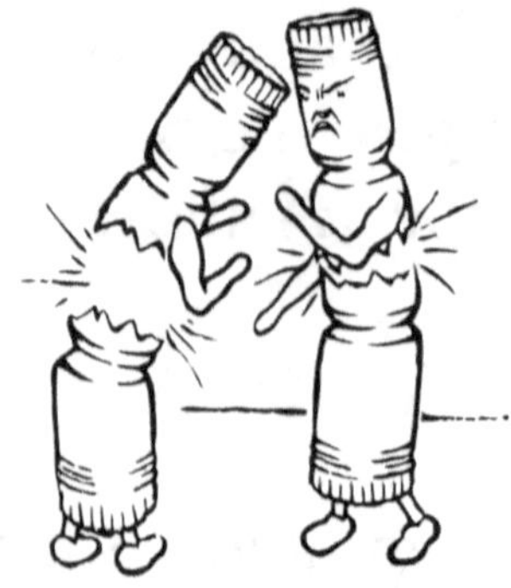

Smokers Fast

Smokers can benefit from a fast on blended organic seeded red grapes with rice bran solubles for seven days. NAC & alpha lipoic acid helps control blood sugar and RBS has high concentrations of this antioxidant. The grapes are able to dissolve mucus in the body very well and added benefits are in grape skins as they contain resveratrol. RBS also contain IP6, tocotrienols, fatty acids, and almost every mineral the body needs. RBS are one of the most complete foods found today, and make a great addition to any cleanse.

Simple Soup Fast

One of my favorite ways to clean the body is by soup fasting. This involves only ingesting blended-only meals such as soups, sherbets, smoothies and vegan yogurts. Blending foods keep insulin and fiber present which brings moisture to the intestines and draws toxins out. Regulation of blood sugar is key to longevity and helping the liver restore itself. Get creative and you will never want to eat solid foods again. Addition of caster packs is amazing with this cleanse.

One can choose to fast on any particular food, but I advise wild grown herbs, fruits or honey. As their superiority over conventionally grown store bought produce cannot be overstated. Today's food, grown in soil missing necessary elements needed for optimal health is not the best for long term consumption, we need to either incorporate a whole-food based multi vitamin/mineral supplement or wild crafted herbs. Whatever you choose to fast on, have an idea on what your purpose and goal is and set a time & strategy for how long you will fast. This gives you time to set aside for rest, contemplation, meditation and focus.

If you are considering becoming more vegetarian or incorporating more vegetables in the diet, consider vegetable juicing along with your regular diet for a few weeks before high consumption of vegetables. As plants have cellulose as their primary cell wall make up, humans have little ability to break down this material. We simply were not designed to consume them to the extent most people are today, thus I recommend vegetable juicing as this removes much of this cellulose & helps the body to more acclimate to these kinds of foods.

Here are two great juice combinations to get you started: celery base with parsley, ginger, turmeric or cayenne; or a cucumber base with added cabbage, celery & pealed de-cored green apple.

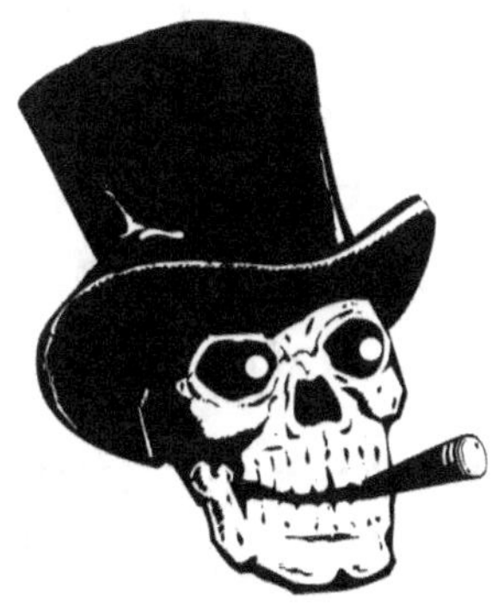

RAW MATT VS. CANCER

This is a controversial topic in the mainstream health community. Sometimes people who are suffering are taken advantage of by those offering "miracle cures."

I am not an allopathic doctor.

I am a simple religious man who has observed God's ways.

If I were to advise a protocol for dealing with cancer, here are some strategies and items that could help you. I would have you ask your doctor about them. If any of them intrigues you, please do more research on them to find out if they are right for you?

- Take protein-digesting enzymes such as protease, papain, pepsin, etc. Take large quantities (such as ten capsules every hour daily) of these for a few months. Viruses, fungi, and other cancer-causing pathogens hide behind protein shells, so destroying the shell will assist your immune system in destroying these pathogens.

- Green hulls of black walnut are a powerful herb that can kill many kinds of parasites that have been linked to cancer.

- Take colloidal silver for ten days, then rest ten days. Consume alone in between meals with no water.

- Eat apricot seeds and milk thistle seeds.

- Take zeolites.

- Do a liver cleanse. It's flush time, follow my previously noted system.

- Try hydrogen peroxide in high-end food grade form. Consume in water, but be careful, if you cannot tolerate HP, add honey (especially Manuka honey UMF 16+) to water and drink, as honey contains high concentrations of HP.

- Guacatonga (casearia sylvestris) contains powerful anti-inflammatory phytochemicals.

- Lactoferrin is immune system kick start.

- Graviola ia a parasite destroyer and immune builder.

- Try Modified Citrus Pectin (MCP).

- The ABM (agaricus blazie murill) mushroom is a known immune system builder from Brazil developed by Japanese Laboratory. It has many positive effects such as arresting tumor growth.

- Spend time around Waterfalls and the ocean!

- Relax and Breath Breath Breath!

- **VERY IMPORTANT:** Consider consuming large doses daily of food-based Vitamin C. (For those who find it too acidic for their stomachs, can be taken as ascorbic acid or in form of ascorbate which will not upset stomach.) Take as much as body will tolerate. Start with 5000 mg. daily, taken throughout the day. If develop a loose stool, decrease by 500 mg. day until stool firm, then keep that amount. Then, work your way back up to 5000 mg. You may safely take any amount of Vitamin C, as there has been no toxicity level shown and it has even been given intravenously in hospitals at doses of 10,000 mg.

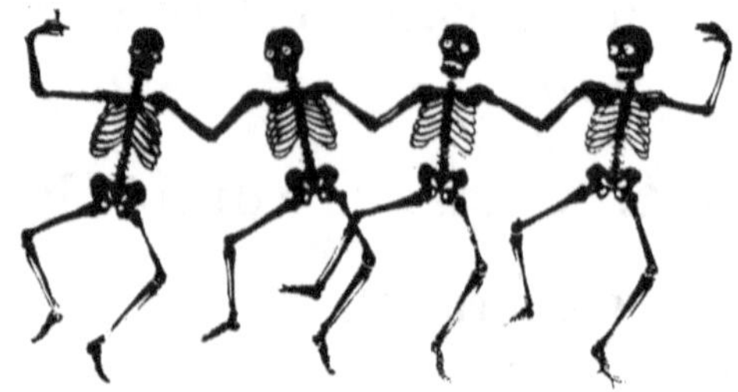

MOVEMENT

Stagnation is never good; we dry up when we don't move. We have three times more lymph than blood, so daily movement is essential to longevity. Rest is different than sitting all day, as rest is an anabolic state that allows muscles to grow and regenerate. We get rest as we sleep, but sitting and believing this is rest does not count.

Sitting is fine, but if your job finds you predominantly sitting all day long, then you must make the time for physical movement/activity or exercise. At a minimum, get onto your feet and stretch every hour for five minutes. If your job allows, get up and do ten minutes of moderate to high-intensity exercise (i.e. sprint intervals, Ashtanga yoga, deadlifts, rowing machine, jumping jacks, jump rope, etc.) every three to four hours. An overweight person who moves will be healthier than someone skinny who does not.

Whatever the activity you might find pleasing whether it be yoga, hiking, martial arts, dancing, running, swimming or any other active sport – just do it! All of these examples are wonderful for the mind body and spirit.

CONCLUSIONS

*"The important thing
is not to stop questioning."*

Albert Einstein

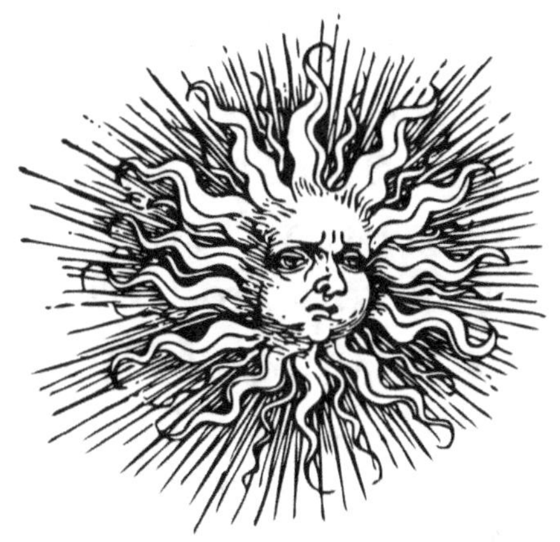

Vibration

We are Light Energy beings vibrating in alignment with our creator. Created by love for love, and until we understand that, fear will reign. Love is more powerful than anything, and can overcome the darkest of dark places. The sun doesn't favor any single blade of grass, but shines upon all equally. We being created by love, share in its power and can manifest any reality we choose for ourselves. Through our mind, we can have a defeatist attitude towards life or an optimistic attitude. When you realize how truly special you are, you can have renewed faith in life itself.

Growth, is letting things go in life that hold you back and bring to your recollection regret. It's the past, and we must realize that there is nothing more we can do to change that past, but look forward to the future. The past is what made you who you are today. So forget living with regret and love where you are at now. Be thankful how truly blessed you are to live at this wonderful time.

The world is always changing, and the only thing constant in life is change.

Motivation

Motivation for changing your diet if you are already "feeling" healthy can be rationalized many different ways. You can look at it from the aspect of your mental health, as your memory greatly improves when diet is modified. Concentration increases and retention of information is greatly increased. Myself, I was diagnosed with ADHD. When in school I was never able to even finish even one book report. Yes, I failed. But after changing my eating habits I found that I was able to sit still and read for hours on end.

Another powerful motivator for diet change would be the aspect of compassion and consciousness for humanity, animals and the earth. The consumption of animal products not only takes the life of a creature, but resources that could have been used to feed other humans are now being fed to animals to feed us. Something like 90% or more of our wheat, corn and rice all go to animals to feed us and literally tons of water! As one doesn't even need to consume meat for health, it is interesting to step back and see the impact your choice to abstain from meat can make on our environment. The number one greenhouse gas causing more pollution than ANY other single source by far is the gas released from factory farms, and their animals.

Aging Can Be Slowed

Another motivator for diet change is the matter of longevity. We age because our bodies weaken from accumulated of byproducts and debris in the body left behind from unhealthy foods. This is one of the main reasons, even though other factors do play a part. But what if the power of Mother Nature was able to sustain us, for extremely long amounts of time? I mean science has shown us that if cells are given the proper nutrition and their waste is removed, they do not die. This is motivation for finding ways to extend life hundreds of years! Truly, some people live to 100 years or more eating pure CRAP! Imagine with the knowledge and foresight we have nowadays and apply that wisdom to everyday life. We should really see a shift in age expectancy and longevity in the near future.

How do I know that the aging process can be slowed dramatically? Well, because it can be sped up! Look at how early kids are going through puberty now a days, in relation to the foods they are eating. Most of the dairy products and meats are pumped full of hormones that obviously have a biological effect on us. Not to mention disease like Werner Syndrome or Progeria translating from Greek to mean "old age". These genetic displacements take effect in children causing them to often age at a superior rate often times losing all their hair by ten years of age or younger. Children with progeria often die in their early teen years of "old age."

The body's internal clock is all regulated by hormonal responses triggered in the brain. Human Growth Hormone (HGH) is produced in the pituitary gland, a small gland at the base of the brain which regulates the endocrine glands. The pituitary is the master glad, regulating the entire hormone system. Almost 50% of the anterior cells are "somatocytes", cells that make HGH. Based on that number of cells nature seems to think that the production of HGH is critically important.

When we are kids we have extra HGH because it is needed in development of bone and final height. At around age 18 the body fuses bone together in direct response to HGH and then levels drop dramatically, since no further lengthening is needed after infusion. Traditionally this is all HGH was thought to do. But modern science shows that every cell in the body has HGH receptors and that it is doing a host of other jobs in every organ of the body and metabolism. There are even receptors in the brain that respond by literally coming back to life. (About 10% of the brains cells become non-functional every 10 years of life). This is why

HGH is the latest and most effective treatment for Alzheimer's disease.

HGH is completely related to aging. When one is on HGH replacement therapy, bone cells respond by making new bone and osteoporosis reverses. Fat cells respond by burning faster and used for energy. Sexual desire increases and hair beings to re-grow. Muscle cells respond by becoming larger and stronger throughout the whole system. Youthful strength and endurance returns, and many can even begin to read without their glasses again. This is apparent that HGH is extremely important factor to the mystery of aging and cannot be overlooked.

As we age HGH seems to dramatically drop, so this is where nutrition comes into play. Fasting helps the body release HGH. Keeping insulin levels down and maintaining blood sugar levels is an important factor in HGH release. Exercising regularly also stimulates HGH. The combining of these three powerful choices and you will find success in true longevity and vitality.

Two of the major glands that play a role in us aging are thyroid and adrenal glands. This is why DHEA became popular. It helps production of these hormones. Diet has a major effect on every aspect of these hormones, how they act in maintaining normal levels of the hormones and maintaining them.

I believe that as we age the worst thing in our life is stress. If one is stressed, cells actually secrete a toxin worse than any chemical ingested. This oxidative stress chemical is called mycotoxin and is viewed through bright field microscopy.

I hope this helps shed some information on this new way to live and eat. The Raw Food diet revolution is not really talked about too much in mainstream media, probably because people are too afraid of losing credibility on such a subject, or being looked at like a nut job. I hope I have evaluated the facts I have discovered with a rational look and without bias. If you have questions about other food, diet and health related topics, I will be available to answer questions on the message board on this site. Because ultimately, it is my wish and desire for you to be informed, be happy, eat well and to have Dominant Health!

APPENDICES

*"Life is like riding a bicycle.
To keep your balance
you must keep moving."*

Albert Einstein

RESOURCES

BodyForce

Effective formulations for parasites, cleansing and weight loss. BodyForceProducts.com

Essenes

Information about the Essene Gospel of Peace. Essene.com and EsseneSchool.com

Libbe Colon Hydrotherapy

Open-system colonics. colonic.net

Lotus Foods

Organic heirloom rice. LotusFoods.com

Mountain Rose Herbs

A great source for organic and wild crafted herbs. MountainRoseHerbs.com

Raw Food Support

Online community that helps raw foodists find each other. rawfoodsupport.com

Vital Choice

If you choose to eat fish, they have a sustainable selection. VitalChoice.com

SELECTED BIBLIOGRAPHY

A.B.R., 'The Old Countess of Desmond' in Notes and Queries1851, p. 305

A.E., Bray, 'The Old Countess of Desmond' in Notes and Queries, 1852, pp.564-565

American Bear Association

Anne Chambers As Wicked a Woman (Dublin, 1986), pp.232-235

augustachronicle.com/stories/060998/fea_graedo.shtml

Caster WO, Burton TA, Irvin TR, Tanner MA. Dietary aflatoxins, intelligence and school performance in southern Georgia. Int J of Vitamin and Nutrition Resource 1986

Chaudhary G, Sharma U, Jagannathan NR, Gupta YK. Evaluation of Withania somnifera in a middle cerebral artery occlusion model of stroke in rats. Clin Exp Pharmacol Physiol. 2003 May-Jun;30(5-6):399-404.

csprosystems.com/BYU_Bacteria_Testing.html Brigham Young University

David A. Revelli, Microbiologist,Dr. Ron W. Leavitt, Ph.D.,Professor of Microbiology/Molecular Biology

Davis L, Kuttan G. Effect of Withania somnifera on CTL activity. J Exp Clin Cancer Res. 2002 Mar;21(1):115-8

Dean and Chapter of Westminster Abbey 2004

demogr.mpg.de/books/odense/6/09.htm

Dictionary of Phrase and Fable, E. Cobham Brewer, 1894

Elmholt, S. (2003)

Ernesto Contreras, M.D., cancer specialist:

Gupta AK, Batra R, Bluhm R, Boekhout T, Dawson TL (2004). "Skin diseases associated with Malassezia species" J. Am. Acad. Dermatol. 51 (5): 785-98. doi:10.1016/j.jaad.2003.12.034. PMID 15523360

Hamilton RD, Foss AJ, Leach L (2007). "Establishment of a human in vitro model of the outer blood-retinal barrier" doi:10.1111/j.1469-7580.2007.00812.x. PMID 17922819

healthtalk.com/go/colitis/disease-basics/10-key-questions-about-ulcerative-colitis?pg=3

Jain S, Shukla SD, Sharma K, Bhatnagar M. Neuroprotective effects of Withania somnifera Dunn. Hippocampal sub-regions of female albino rat. Phytother Res. 2001 Sep;15(6):544-8.

jama.ama-assn.org/cgi/content/full/285/24/3093

Journal of American Science, 3(3), 2007, Ma Hongbao, Horng Dengnan, Cherng Shen, Colloidal Silver

Junqueira, L.C.; J. Carneiro. Basic Histology: Text and Atlas, 10th ed. (Statistic page 161)

KJV Matthew_3:4 (about john the baptist)

Knox, Angie (June 8, 2004), Harnessing honey's healing power, news.bbc.co.uk/1/hi/health/3787867.stm Retrieved on June 2, 2007

Kuboyama T, Tohda C, Zhao J, Nakamura N, Hattori M, Komatsu K. Axon- or dendrite-predominant outgrowth induced by constituents from Ashwagandha. Neuroreport. 2002 Oct 7;13(14):1715-20

latimes.com/pulitzer

ncbi.nlm.nih.gov/pubmed/16880289 & ncbi.nlm.nih.gov/pubmed/7784468

Noens I, van Berckelaer-Onnes I, Verpoorten R, van Duijn G (2006). "The ComFor: an instrument for the indication of augmentative communication in people with autism and intellectual disability". J Intellect Disabil Res 50 (9): 621–32

northstar-website-design.com/resources/old_parr.html

Ochratoxin A and Aflatoxins found at http://www.helica.com/home/

Parihar MS, Hemnani T.Phenolic antioxidants attenuate hippocampal neuronal cell damage against kainic acid induced excitotoxicity. J Biosci. 2003 Feb;28(1):121-8.

Qur'an 47:15 and Translation of Quran 16:68-69

Rang, H. P. (2003). Pharmacology. Edinburgh: Churchill Livingstone, page 474 for noradrenaline system, page 476 for dopamine system, page 480 for serotonin system and page 483 for cholinergic system.. ISBN 0-443-07145-4

Sahih Bukhari vol. 7, book 69, number 504 and 518

Sigmund Schmidt, M.D., The Natural Health Clinic, Bad Bothenfelds

time.com/time/magazine/article/0,9171,745510,00.html

Tohda C, Kuboyama T, Komatsu K. Dendrite extension by methanol extract of Ashwagandha (roots of Withania somnifera) in SK-N-SH cells. Neuroreport. 2000 Jun 26;11(9):1981-5

"Tortoise-Pigeon-Dog" Article From the May 15, 1933 issue of Time magazine

Venerable Archdeacon A. B. Rowan, The Olde Countess of Desmond: her Identitie; her Portraiture; her Descente in The Dublin Review, vol. LI [1862], p. 51

Vugler A, Lawrence J, Walsh J, et al (2007). "Embryonic stem cells and retinal repair" doi:10.1016/j.mod.2007.08.002. PMID 17881192

Wahdan H. "Causes of the antimicrobial activity of honey". Infection 26 (1): 26-31. PMID 9505176

webmd.com/digestive-disorders/tc/clostridium-difficile-colitis-overview

westminster-abbey.org/history-research/monuments-gravestones/people/12190

zeoliteautismstudy.com/home/index.php?option=com_frontpage&Itemid=1

Epic Elixirs

At one point I produced elixirs with super-foods suspended in unheated unprocessed honey. I called them "Epic Elixirs."

Here are a couple of my formulas you can try to make:

- Immortality ~ goji, mesquite, fo-ti, vanilla

- Beauty ~ cacao, fo-ti, milk thistle, lucuma

- Ecstasy ~ coconut, lucuma, cacao, cayenne

I encourage you to experiment making your own synergistic elixir combinations. Here are some tips on dealing with honey.

See if you can find a local bee keeper to work with and make sure the bees are well taken care of. Honey should never see the light of day. Keep it stored in a dark place. When honey remains in direct sunlight for about one day, its lysozyme (antibacterial albuminous enzyme) is destroyed. Raw honey may also contain pollen and royal jelly which are destroyed by light and heat. Honey should also be protected from oxygen, which accelerates crystallization.

SOME OF MY FAVORITE HERBS

You are advised to store all herbs in glass jar out of light in a cool temperature.

Artichoke

Artichoke has been used in traditional medicine for centuries as a specific liver and gallbladder remedy. In Brazilian herbal medicine systems, leaf preparations are used for liver and gallbladder problems, diabetes, high cholesterol, hypertension, anemia, diarrhea (and elimination in general), fevers, ulcers, and gout. In Europe, it is also used for liver and gallbladder disorders with tons of research behind it.

Boerhavia Diffusa (aka erva tostao)

G. L. Cruz, one of Brazil's leading medical herbalists, reports erva tostão is "a plant medicine of great importance, extraordinarily beneficial in the treatment of liver disorders." It is employed in Brazilian herbal medicine to stimulate the emptying of the gallbladder, as a diuretic, for all types of liver disorders (including jaundice and hepatitis), gallbladder pain and stones, urinary tract disorders, renal disorders, kidney stones, cystitis, and nephritis. In Ayurvedic herbal medicine systems in India, the roots are employed as a diuretic, digestive aid, laxative, and menstrual promoter and to treat gonorrhea, internal inflammation of all kinds, edema, jaundice, menstrual problems, anemia, and liver, gallbladder, and kidney disorders.

Boldo

In American herbal medicine systems, boldo leaf is used to stimulate the secretion of saliva, bile flow and liver activity; it's chiefly valued as a remedy for gallstones, liver problems, and gallbladder pain.

Burdock Root

Burdock root appears to prevent liver damage caused by alcohol, chemicals, or medications. The exact reason for this protective effect is not known, but it is thought to involve opposition of a chemical process called oxidation, which occurs in the body. One result of oxidation is the release of oxygen free radicals, natural chemicals that may suppress immune function. Antioxidants such as burdock root may protect body cells from damage caused by oxidation.

Chanca Piedra

The Spanish name of the plant, chanca piedra, means "stone breaker" or "shatter stone." It was named for its effective use to generations of Amazonian indigenous peoples in eliminating gallstones and kidney stones. Its main uses are for many types of biliary and urinary conditions including kidney and gallbladder stones; for hepatitis, colds, flu, tuberculosis, and other viral infections; liver diseases and disorders including anemia, jaundice and liver cancer

Dandelion Root

The dandelion has two particularly important uses. One, to promote the formation of bile and to remove excess water from the body in edema conditions resulting from liver problems. By acting to remove poisons from the body, it acts as a tonic and stimulant. The fresh juice is most effective, but dandelion is also prepared as a tea. An infusion of the fresh root is said to be good for gallstones, jaundice, and other liver problems.

Milk Thistle

Milk thistle has protective effects on the liver and to greatly improve its function. It is typically used to treat liver cirrhosis, chronic hepatitis (liver inflammation), and gallbladder disorders. The active compound in Milk thistle is silymarin. You can obtain milk thistle at most health food stores today, use it to make nut milk or grind into powder and take a tablespoons twice a day.

Turmeric

The active compound in turmeric is curcumin, powerful Antioxidant anti-tumor antioxidant, anti-arthritic, anti-amyloid, anti-ischemic and anti-inflammatory properties. Anti-inflammatory properties may be due to inhibition of eicosanoid biosynthesis. In addition it may be effective in treating malaria, prevention of cervical cancer, and may interfere with the replication of the HIV virus. For its optimal potency it needs to be used in conjunction with piperine (extracted from black pepper). This combo makes it 2000 times stronger!

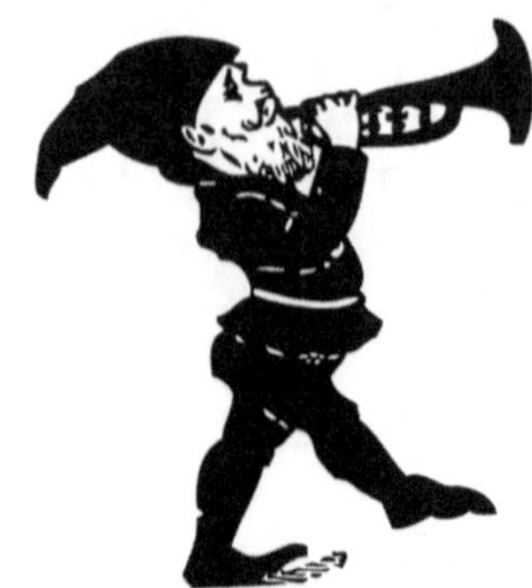

ABOUT THE AUTHOR

At the age of seventeen, Matthew began his fruitful career as a professional fighter winning numerous competitions in the King of Cage I, II, and III, Gladiator Challenge 8, Rage in the Cage, and Mat Madness. He also competed and won in a prominent Jujitsu purple belt competition in Brazil. Shortly thereafter, he began operating Fight Sport in southern California, educating aspiring fighters in the art of Brazilian Jujitsu, Muay, Thai, and Judo.

After a conversation over a sandwich in 2002, Matt became a raw foodist while still professionally fighting. Since that time, he has dedicated much of his time to seeking out health, dietary, and spiritual knowledge. He became an ordained Essene minister and experimented with many dietary protocols including fruitarianism, fasting, breatharianism, liquidarianism, and the typical fat-laden raw food diet. During one eight month experiment, he exclusively ate raw honey that he wild harvested himself.

Over the past several years he developed delicious raw food recipes that have been featured in best-selling books by Dr. Craig Sommers and Dr. David Jubb. Given free lectures all over the West Coast, and created formulations for the successful natural product line by Markus Productions including BodyForce Parasite-Free.

In 2008 he spent nine months in the jungles of Kuai, living exclusively off the land as Nature intended. Immediately on his return, he began lecturing and writing once more, determined to continue helping people improve their lives, including a personal project called, Epic Elixirs, with wild honey and herb formulas that repeatedly sold out in stores.

Matthew is avidly interested in the benefits of bee products and practical applications and scientific studies on physical immortality and the real causes for aging. Time does not age us. Our choices age us.

The Way

End notes by ~anand

"The consumption of animal flesh was unknown up until the great flood. But since the great flood, we have had animal flesh stuffed into our mouths. Jesus, the Christ, who appeared when the time was fulfilled, again joined the end to the beginning, so that we are now no longer allowed to eat animal flesh."

(early church father Eusebius Hieronymus aka Saint Jerome)

For those interested in understanding the theological basis for Matt's diet, please read the Bible. Here are some of his favorite of many quotes in the Old Testament regarding either animals being sacred to G*d or about vegetarianism:

Genesis 1:29-30, Job 12:7, Exodus 20:13, Exodus 23: 12, Exodus 26:34, Leviticus 17:10, Isaiah 65, Isaiah 66:3, Daniel 1, Psalm 50:10, Proverbs 12:10, and Ecclesiastes 3:19

In the New Testament, Yeshua (meaning Salvation - more commonly known by his incorrect Latin-Greek era name, Jesus, from Ie-Sous meaning "Hail Zeus!") was a strict follower of Jewish dietary law as outlined in the Torah. Meaning… He ate Kosher. If you are a true follower of Christ, then at the very least, you should be eating by strict Jewish Kosher rules. It is sad that the early church had such a harsh rejection of Jewish practices, when in fact, Yeshua was a Jewish rabbi whose mission was to bring the Good News to HIS (Jewish) people.

Unlike the Old Testament which had a tradition of native-tongue Aramaic and Hebrew scripture, the New Testament has shortcomings, inclusions, omissions and translation issues due to it telling an Aramaic story in Greek which was translated to Latin and eventually English. This is compounded by the fancies of the early Church leaders up to the printing of the Gutenberg Bible. In the 1500s a scholar named Erasmus who later produced a Greek New Testament criticized the Gutenberg Latin translations and even wrote to his Pope that he had personally 'improved' upon the original Greek text!

Yeshua may have multiplied the loaves and 'pickled' fish, for the people gathered to hear Him speak, but He was not specifically recorded as ever eating that fish. And if the Last Supper was a Passover meal, I attended a vegetarian Seder once and it was delightful. Later in the New Testament, after His resurrection, He was offered broiled fish. Once again we have a convenient mis-translation and even complete omission of the original Greek in some translations of the bible. Yeshua was offered fish AND honeycomb. He took "it," not "them" both.

The original followers of Yeshua were known as "The Way" from the continuation of Yeshua's saying, "'I AM [is] the Way…" Converts were known as proselytes who accepted the doctrines and precepts of Jewish ways. When later evangelists Paul and the 'rejected' apostle Barnabas went to spread the Good News to the Gentiles, they become known as "Christians."

'Saint' Paul (who had never even met Yeshua) decided that two specific parts of His teaching (circumcision and eating clean) were not essential teachings to share. While the early members of The Way allowed circumcision to go by the wayside, they believed strongly in the correct Way of eating that Yeshua had taught them. It was a matter of having reverence for all of G*d's creations and as per the book of Genesis ~ being a conscious steward, not a killer nor eater, of all His treasured creatures.

Paul argues in his epistles against the original disciples (especially against the apostles James, Peter, and John, who HAD known and eaten with Yeshua) about what was clean and unclean food. It is believed that Paul did this to increase the popularity of his version of Christianity. It was a lot easier to gain converts if they could continue to eat meat and be saved by faith alone and not by actual actions! When you become familiar with Yeshua's teaching, you know that He sacrificed Himself as the Passover Lamb as our penance, and so that animals would ever need to be sacrificed again.

G*d gave His beloved humans the perfect raw veganic diet in the Garden of Eden. Please check out our friend Cherry Capri's book, <u>Eat Like Eve</u>, where my husband and I developed many delicious recipes for this Garden of Eden type diet.

www.ingramcontent.com/pod-product-compliance
Lightning Source LLC
Chambersburg PA
CBHW050906260726
48660CB00001B/51